Anatomy Muscular System Label Practice

By K.R. Lefkowitz

Copyright © 2016 K.R. Lefkowitz

All rights reserved.

ISBN: 10:1532996780
ISBN-13: 978-1532996788

MUSCULAR SYSTEM

1. ABDOMINAL M - DEEP
2. ABDOMINAL M - SUPERFICIAL
3. ANKLE & FOOT - TENDONS
4. ANTERIOR MUSCLES - SUPERFICIAL
5. ARM MUSCLES - SUPERFICIAL
6. ARM MUSCLES - SUPERFICIAL 2
7. ARM MUSCLES 1
8. ARM MUSCLES 2
9. ARM MUSCLES 3
10. BACK & NECK MUSCLES - DEEP
11. BACK MUSCLES - SUPERFICIAL
12. BONES & LIGAMENTS - ANKLES
13. BONES & LIGAMENTS - ELBOW 1
14. BONES & LIGAMENTS - ELBOW 2
15. BONES & LIGAMENTS - FOREARM
16. BONES & LIGAMENTS - KNEE 1
17. BONES & LIGAMENTS - KNEE 2
18. BONES & LIGAMENTS - NECK
19. BONES & LIGAMENTS - PELVIS
20. BONES & LIGAMENTS - SPINE
21. CORACOBRACHIAL & BRACHIAL
22. DELTOID MUSCLE
23. DISSECTION - DORSUM OF FOOT
24. DISSECTION - HAND SUPERFICIAL
25. DISSECTION - PALM, INTERMED
26. DISSECTION - PALM SUPERFICIAL
27. FOOT MUSCLES - SUPERFICIAL
28. FOREARM - GENERAL
29. FOREARM - SUPERFICIAL EXT
30. FOREARM - SUPERFICIAL FLEXORS
31. FOREARM M - DEEP EXTENSORS
32. FOREARM M - DEEP FLEXORS
33. FOREARM M - DEEP
34. FOREARM M - SUPERFICIAL 1
35. FOREARM M - SUPERFICIAL 2
36. HAND - DEEP MUSCLES
37. HAND M - LUMBRICAL
38. HAND MUSCLES - SUPERFICIAL
39. HIP & THIGH MUSCLES - DEEP
40. HIP MUSCLES - SUPERFICIAL 1
41. HIP MUSCLES - SUPERFICIAL 2
42. KNEE - MUSCLES & TENDONS 1
43. KNEE - MUSCLES & TENDONS 2
44. KNEE - MUSCLE & TENDONS 3
45. KNEE MUSCLES
46. LEG MUSCLES - EXTENSORS
47. LEG MUSCLES - PERINEAL
48. LEG MUSCLES - SUPERFICIAL 1
49. LEG MUSCLES - SUPERFICIAL 2
50. LEG MUSCLES - SUPERFICIAL 3
51. LEG MUSCLES - SUPERFICIAL 4
52. LEG MUSCLES - SUPERFICIAL 5
53. LEG MUSCLES - PLANTAR FLEX
54. LUMBAR SPINE LIGAMENTS
55. M OF FACIAL EXPRESSION
56. MUSCLES - SUPERFICIAL 1
57. MUSCLES - SUPERFICIAL 2
58. MUSCLES - SUPERFICIAL 3
59. MUSCLES - SUPERFICIAL 4
60. MUSCLES - SUPERFICIAL 5
61. NECK MUSCLES INTERMEDIATE
62. NECK MUSCLES - SUPERFICIAL 1
63. NECK MUSCLES SUPERFICIAL 2
64. PECTORAL GIRDLE

65. QUADRICEPS FEMORIS MUSCLES
66. SCAPULAR MUSCLES
67. SERRATES ANTERIOR MUSCLE
68. TENDON ATTACH - FINGER 1
69. TENDON ATTACH - FINGER 2
70. THIGH MUSCLES - DEEP
71. THIGH MUSCLES - SUPERFICIAL
72. THORACIC MUSCLES - DEEP
73. THORAX & SHOULDER MUSCLES
74. TRICEP MUSCLE

How To Use....

This book is mean't to be used for you to label and practice the components of the cardiovascular system. In going through your anatomy class and later in medical field you will need to know how to label the components, pictures of each system and know it inside and out. The best way is for you to label all the components that you know yourself and research the areas that you don't. Can you label all parts of the heart, ventricles, parties, veins, etc...? Can you recognize a picture and know immediately what it is? You can find the corresponding picture in the table of contents. Nothing is labeled on purpose. This is for you to label. For you to know. And what you don't know for you to research in your texts and find the answers. Through this way of learning and researching the parts you don't know, allows you to actually learn it and have it stored in long term memory. This active way of learning will in the long term be beneficial beyond belief in your future career or knowledge. Mark the pages, make notes, and use this practice book and pictures to help you understand the parts of the anatomy.

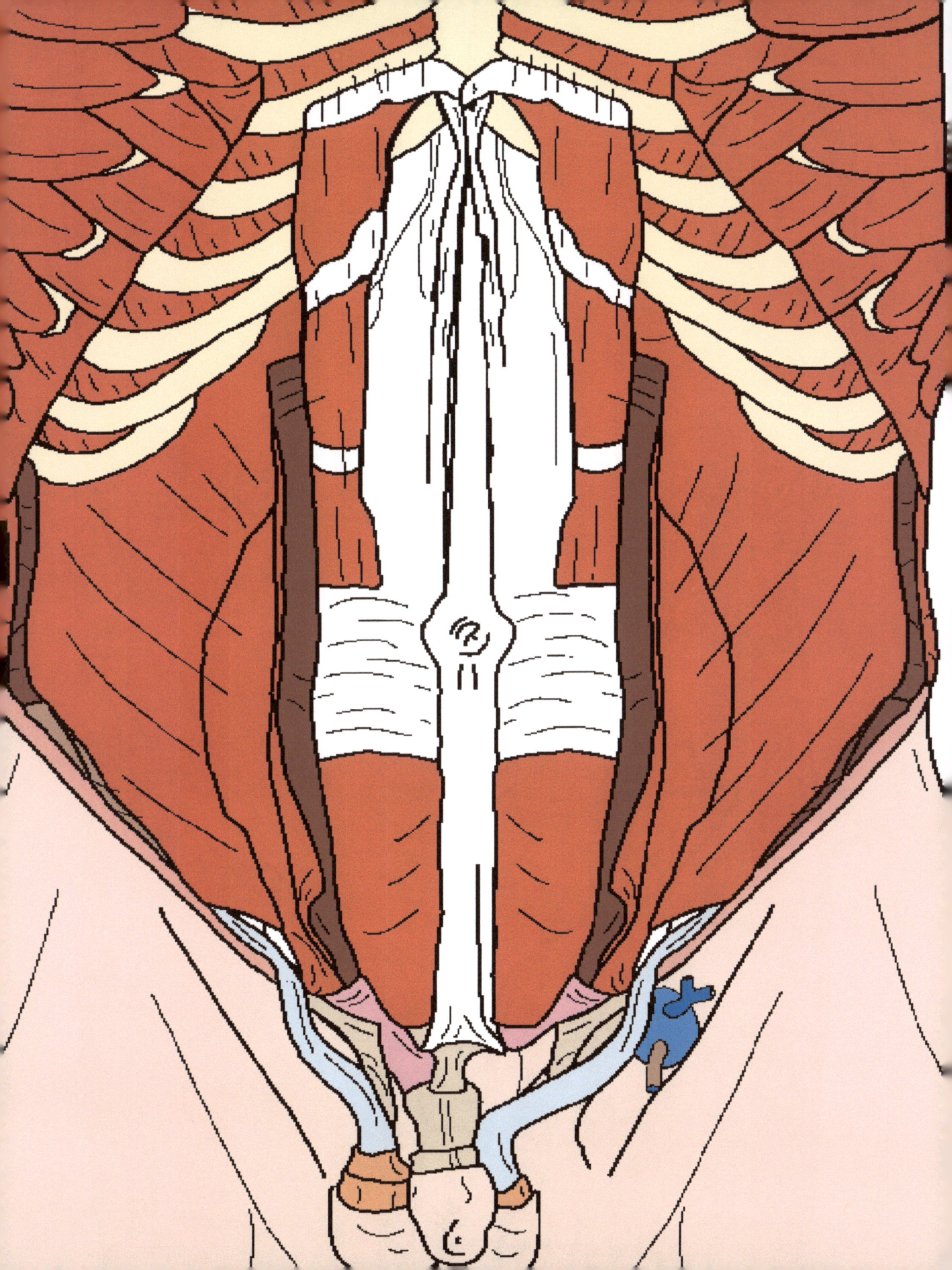

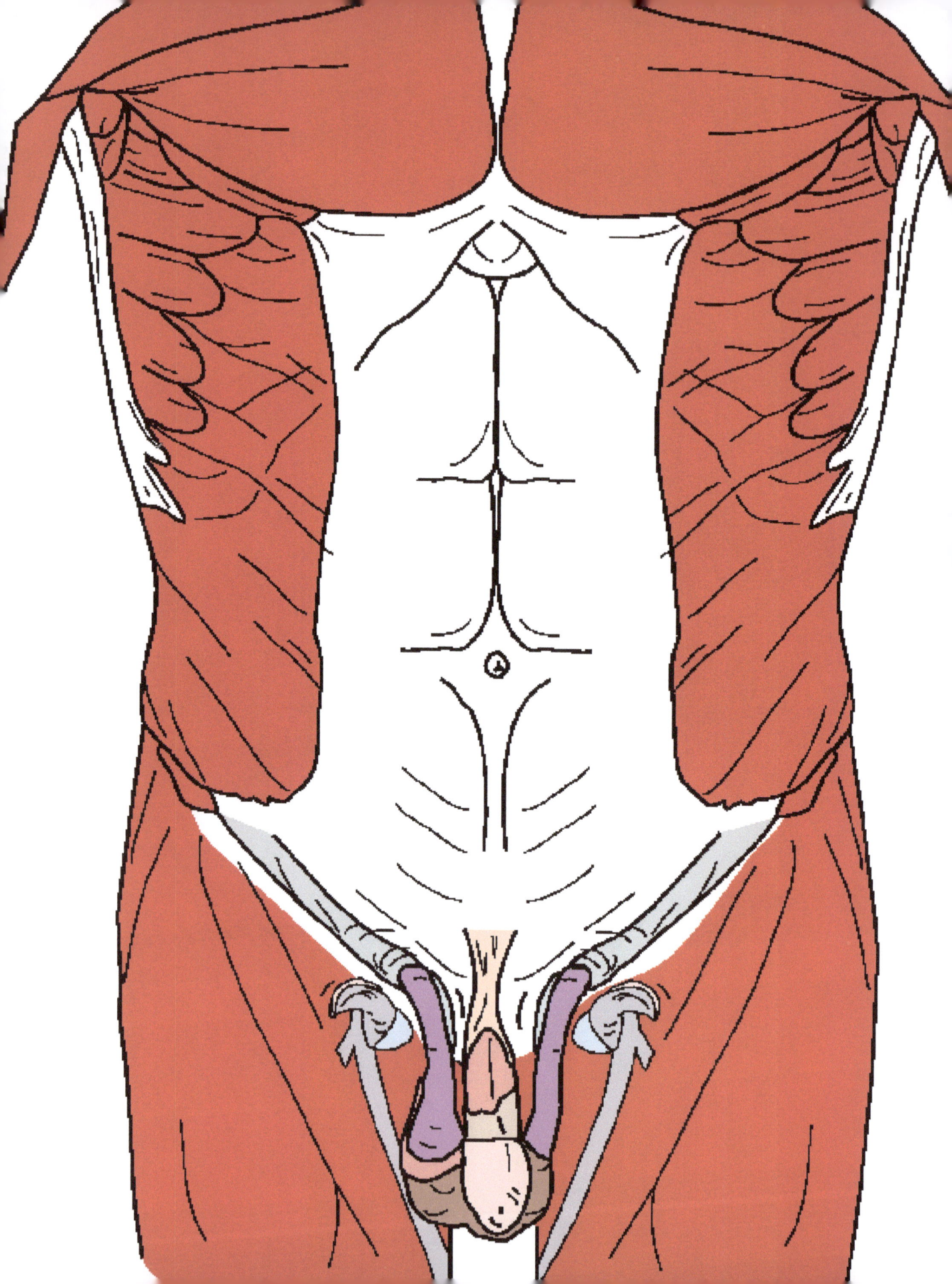

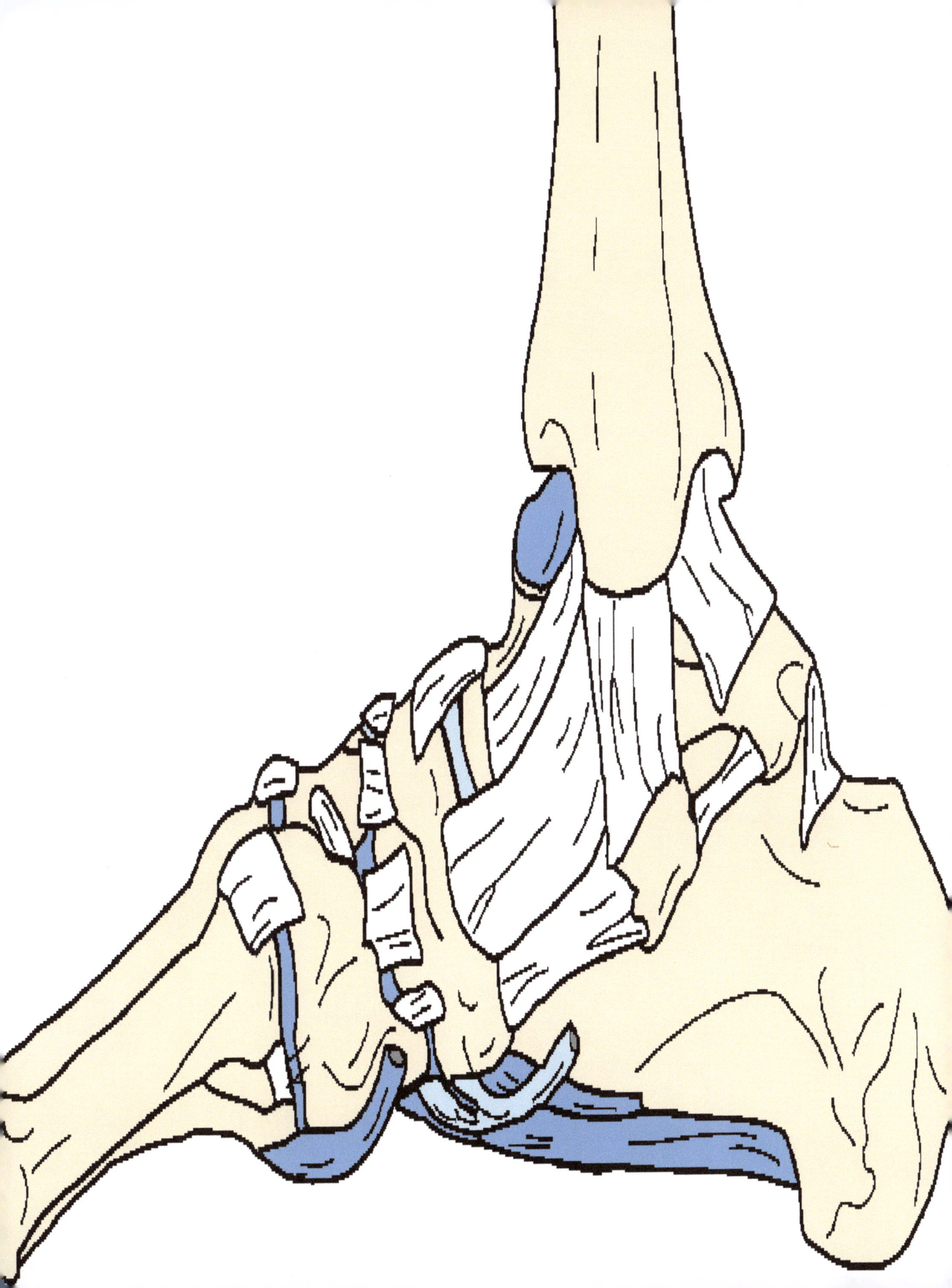

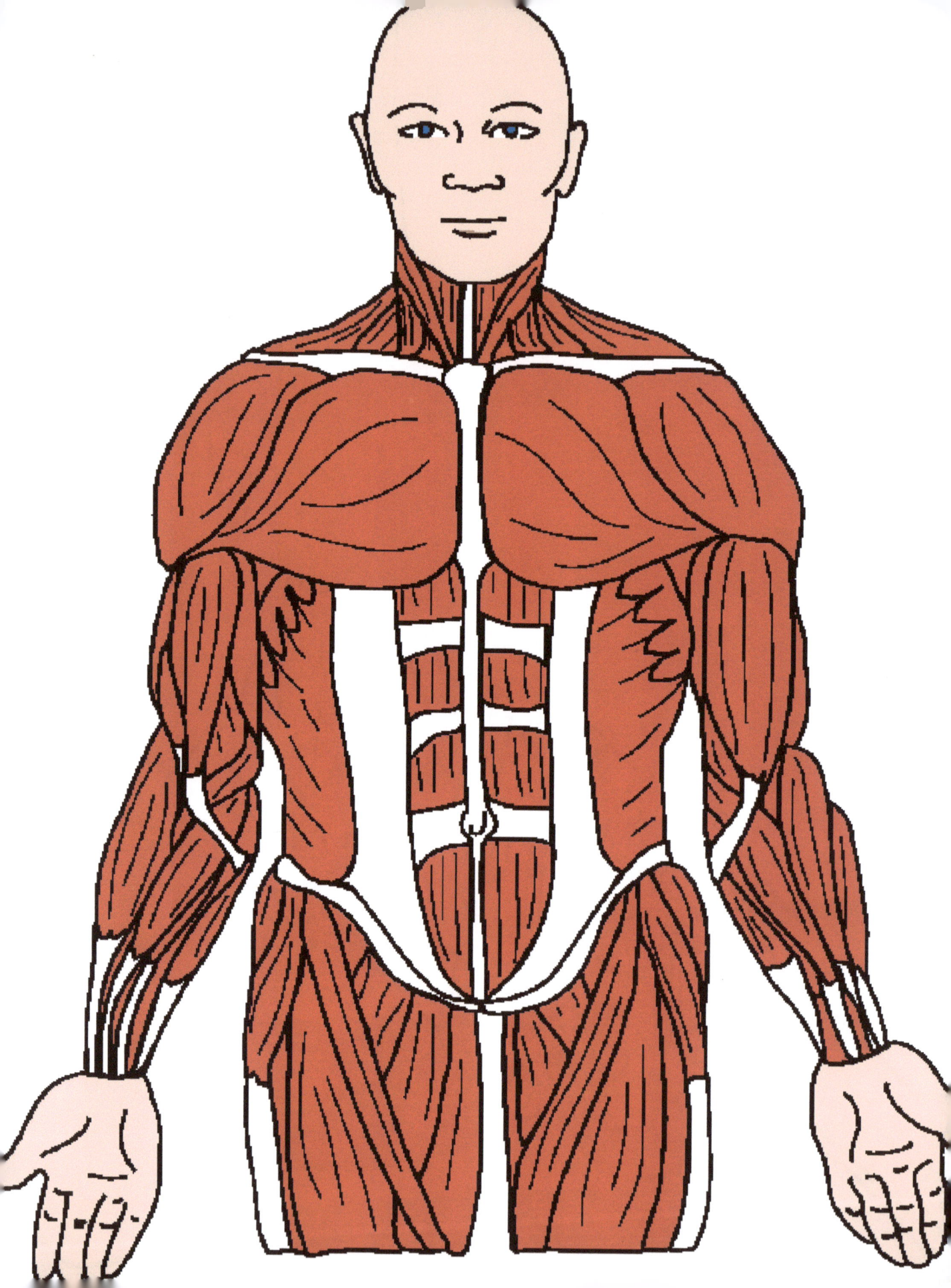

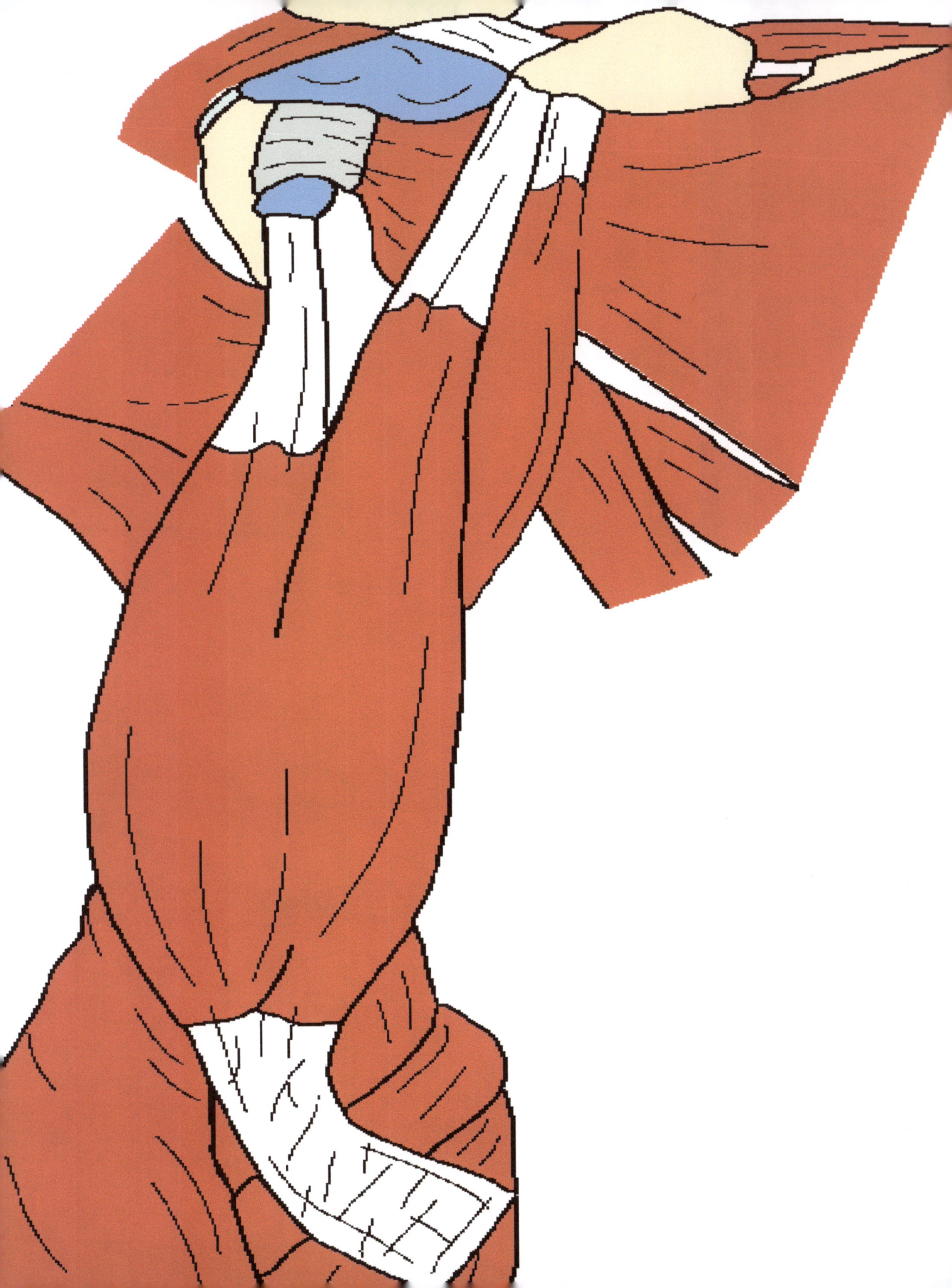

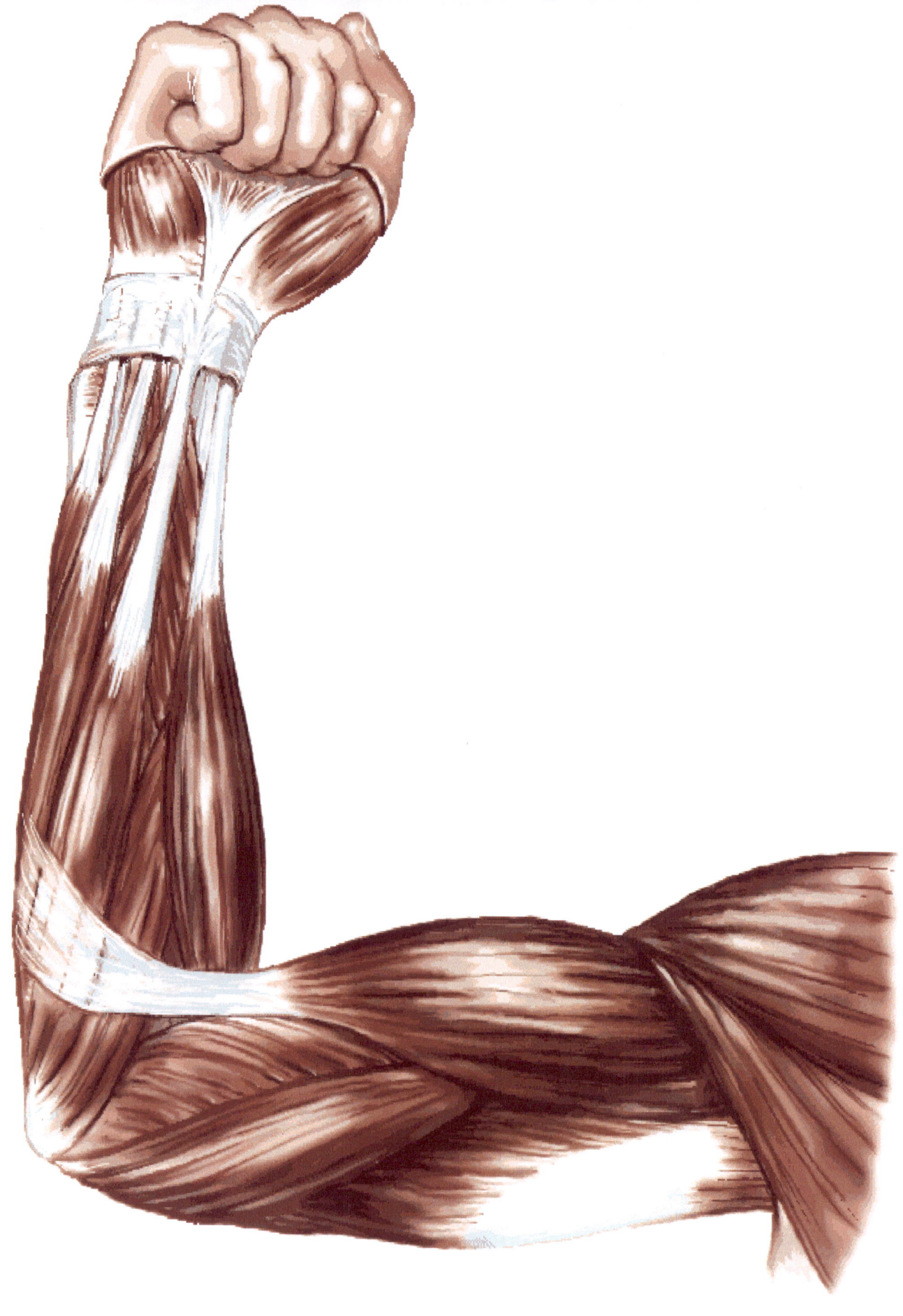

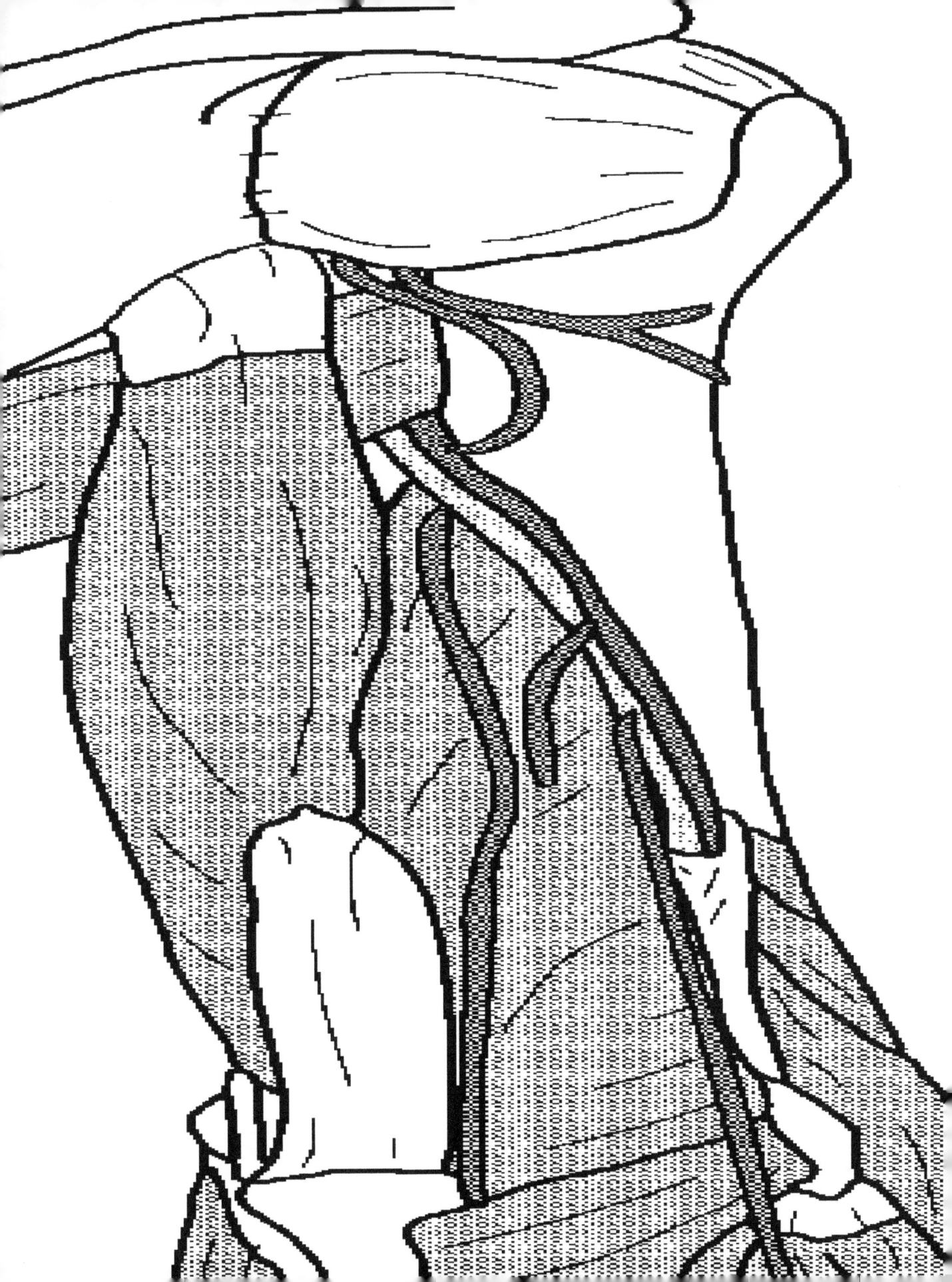

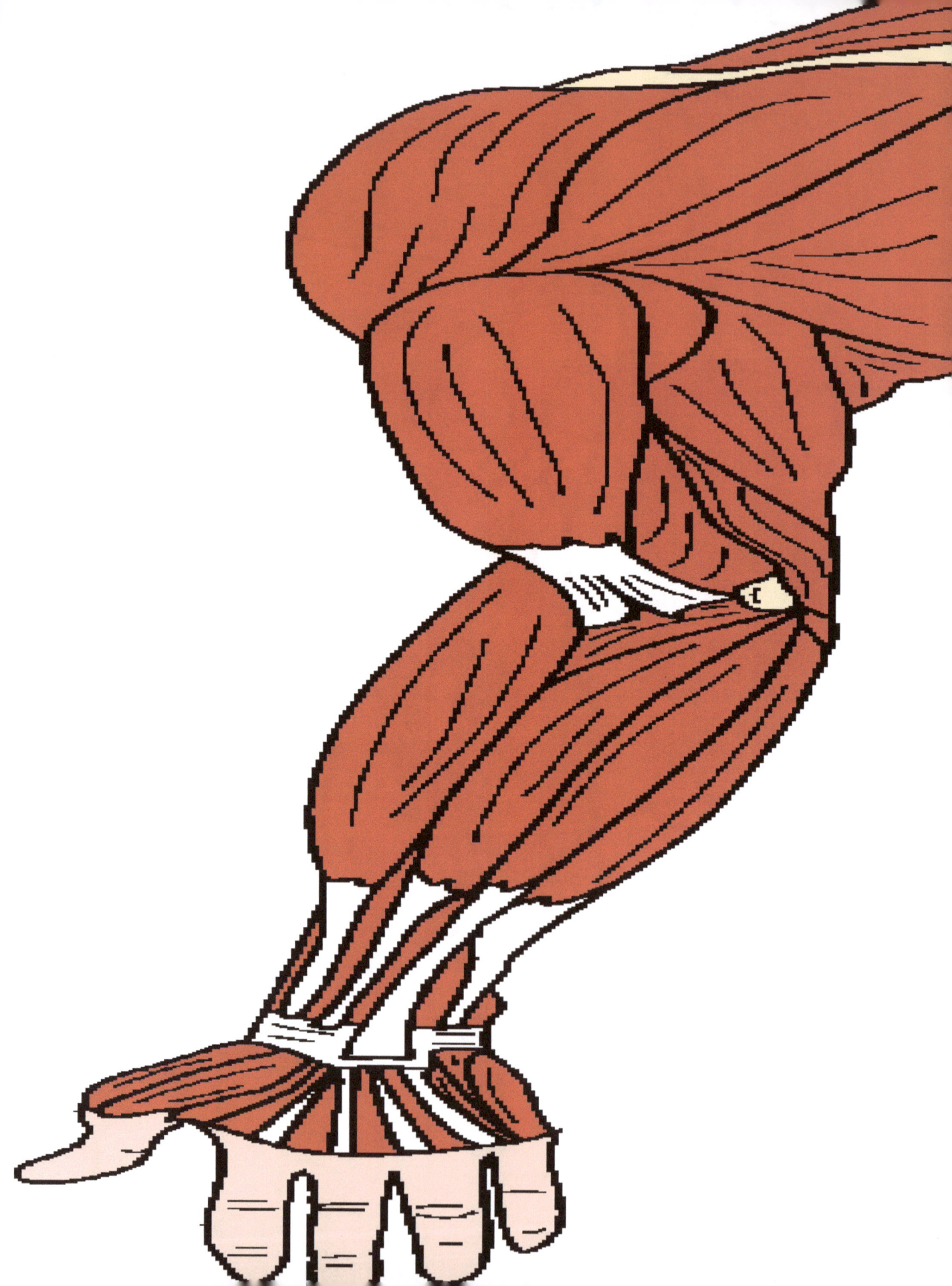

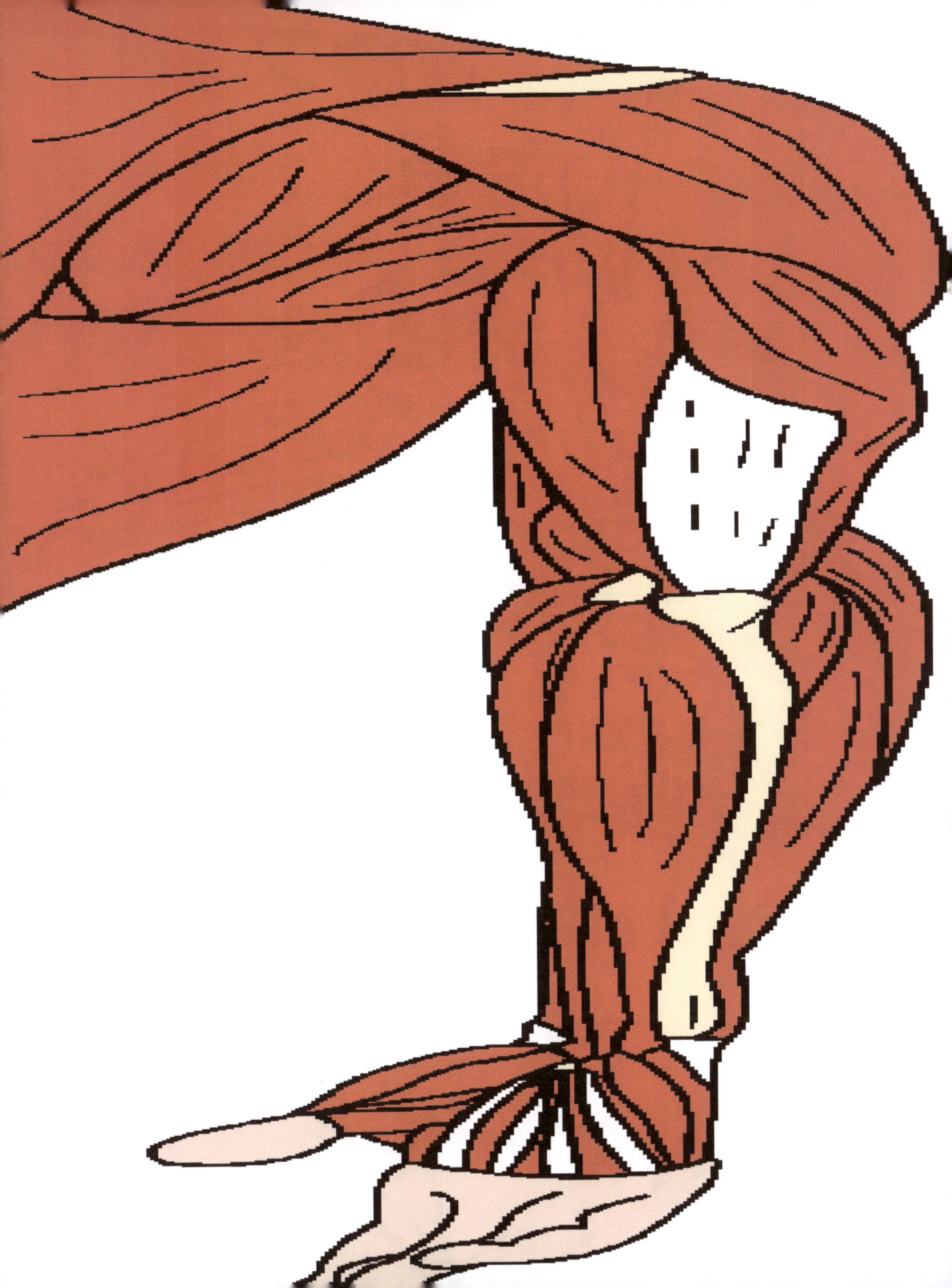

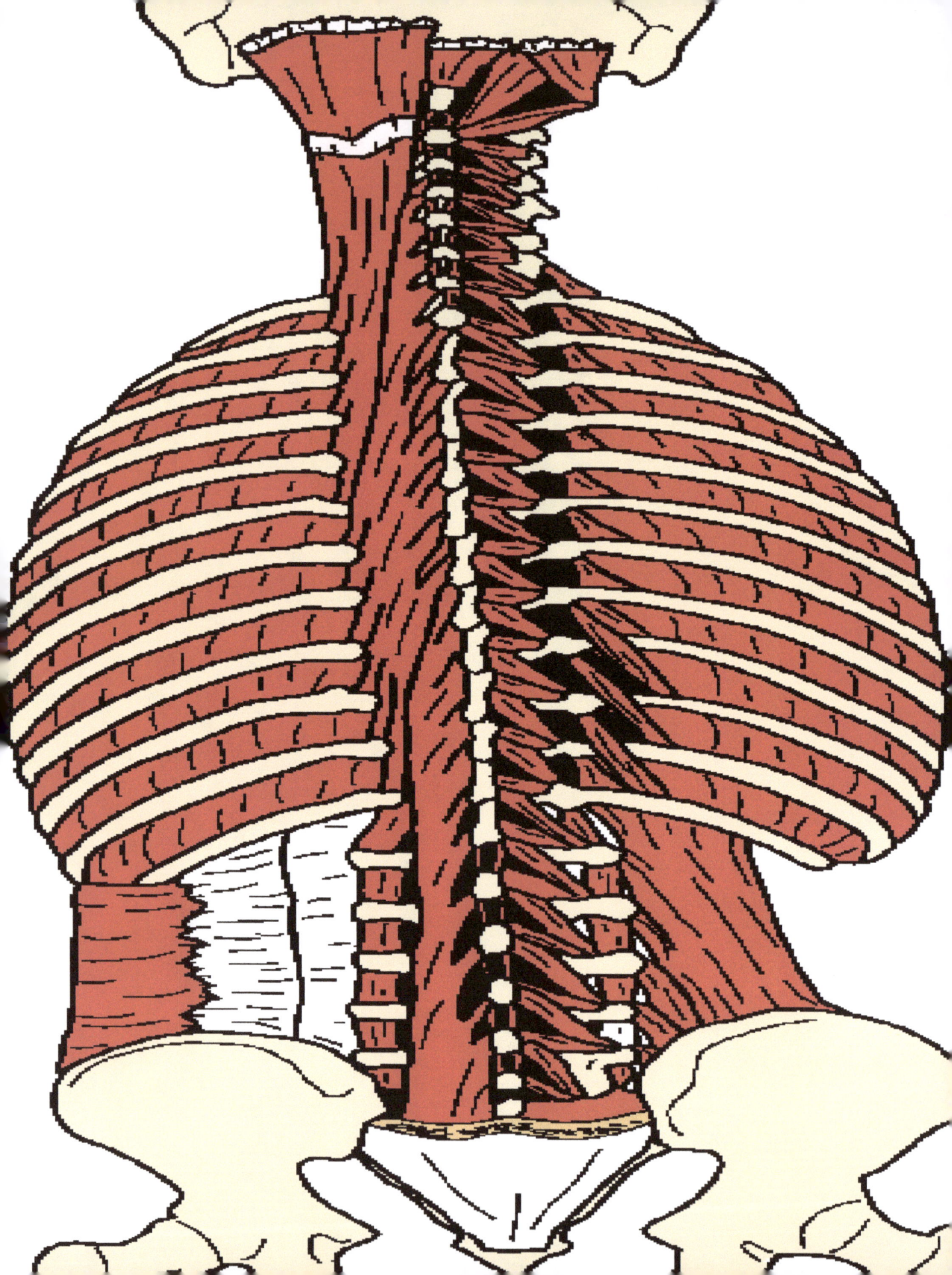

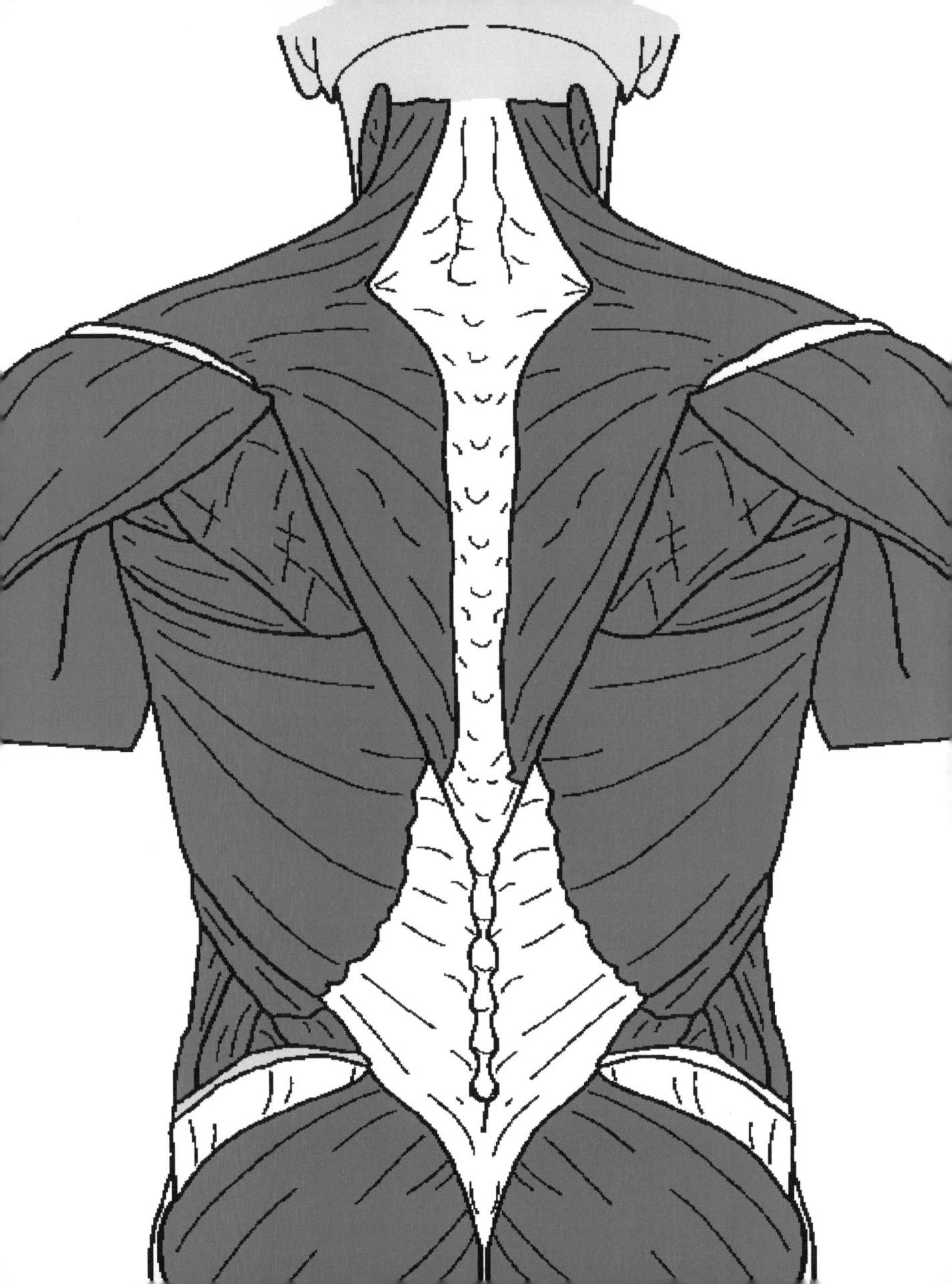

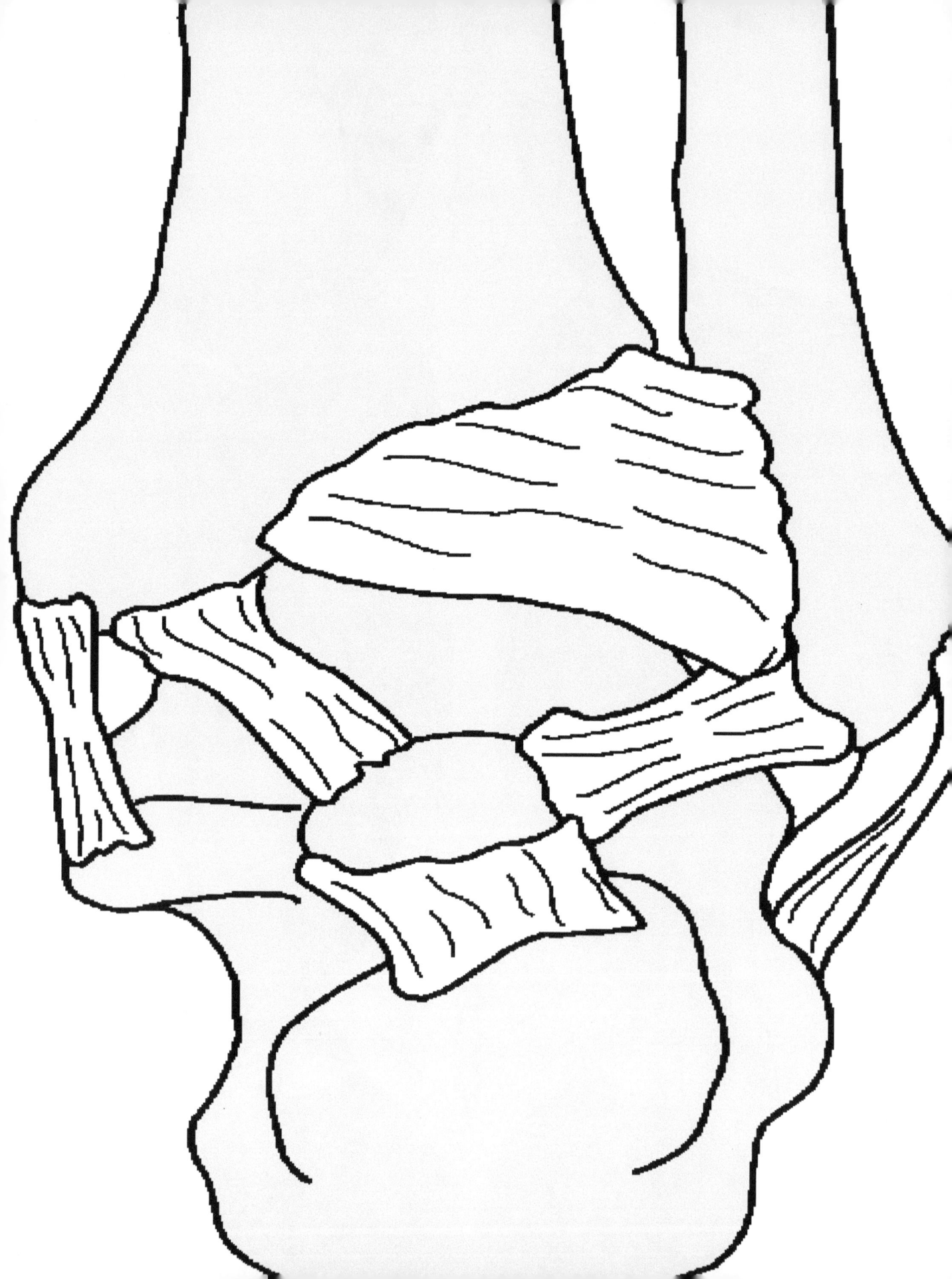

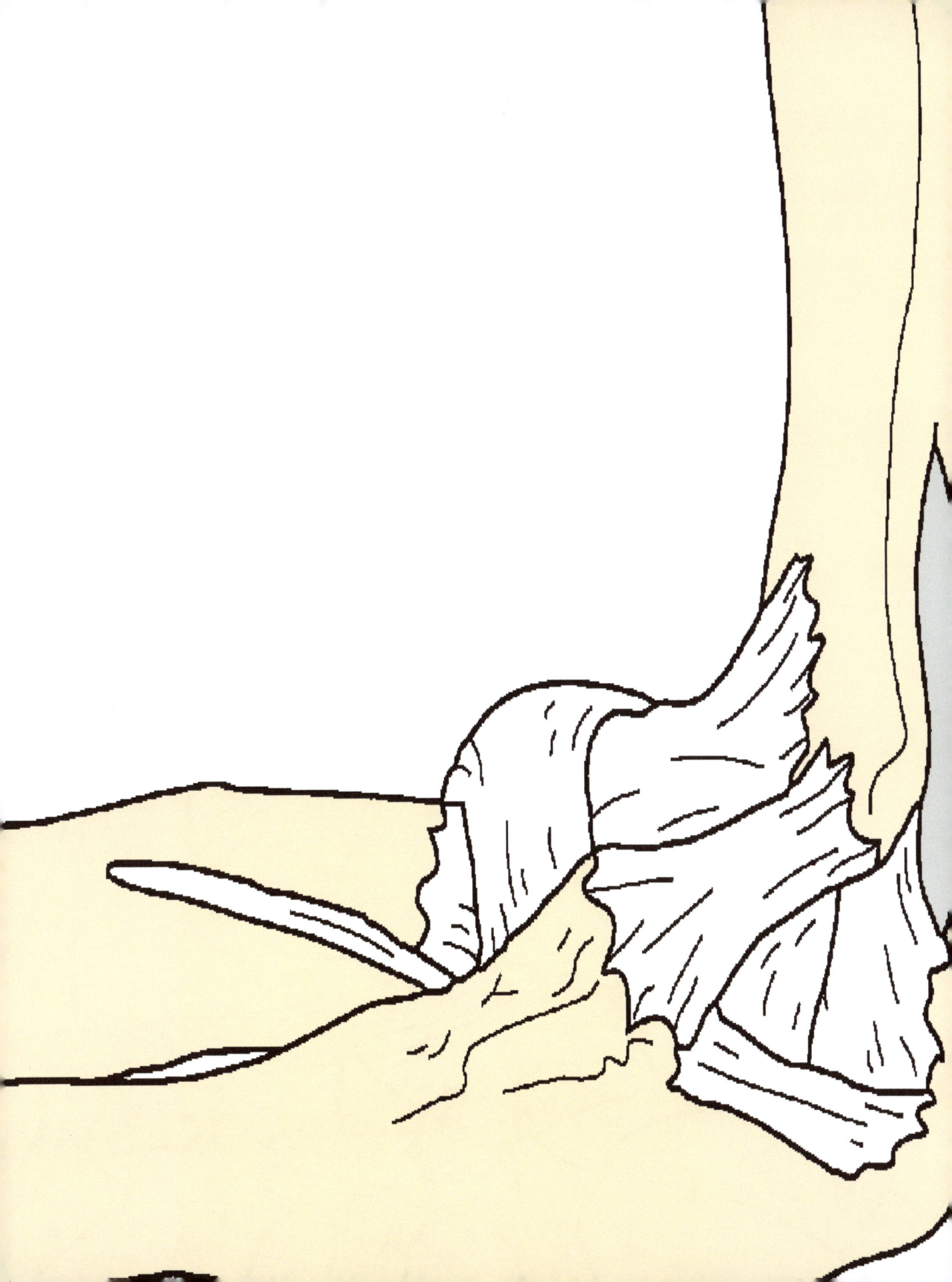

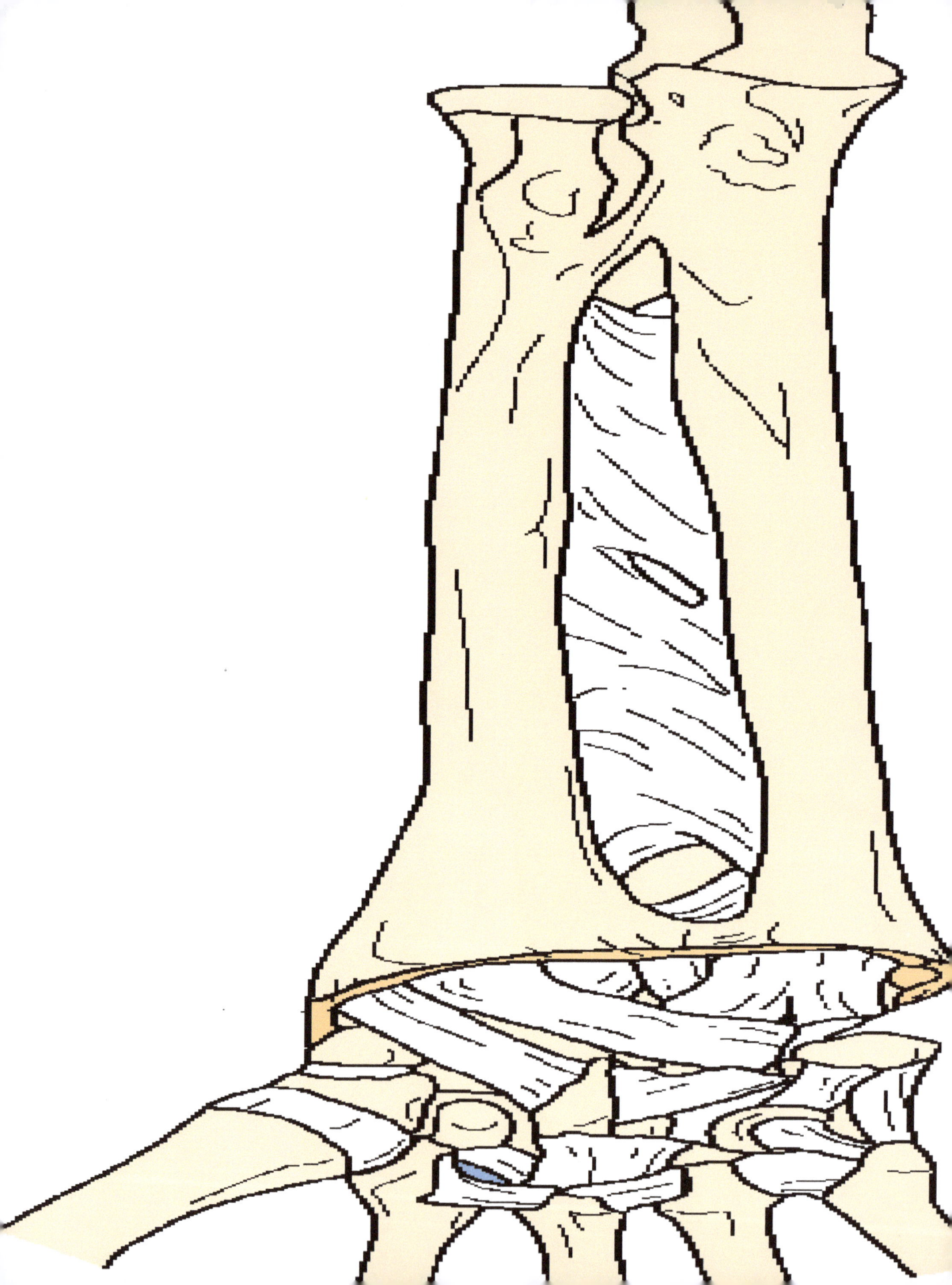

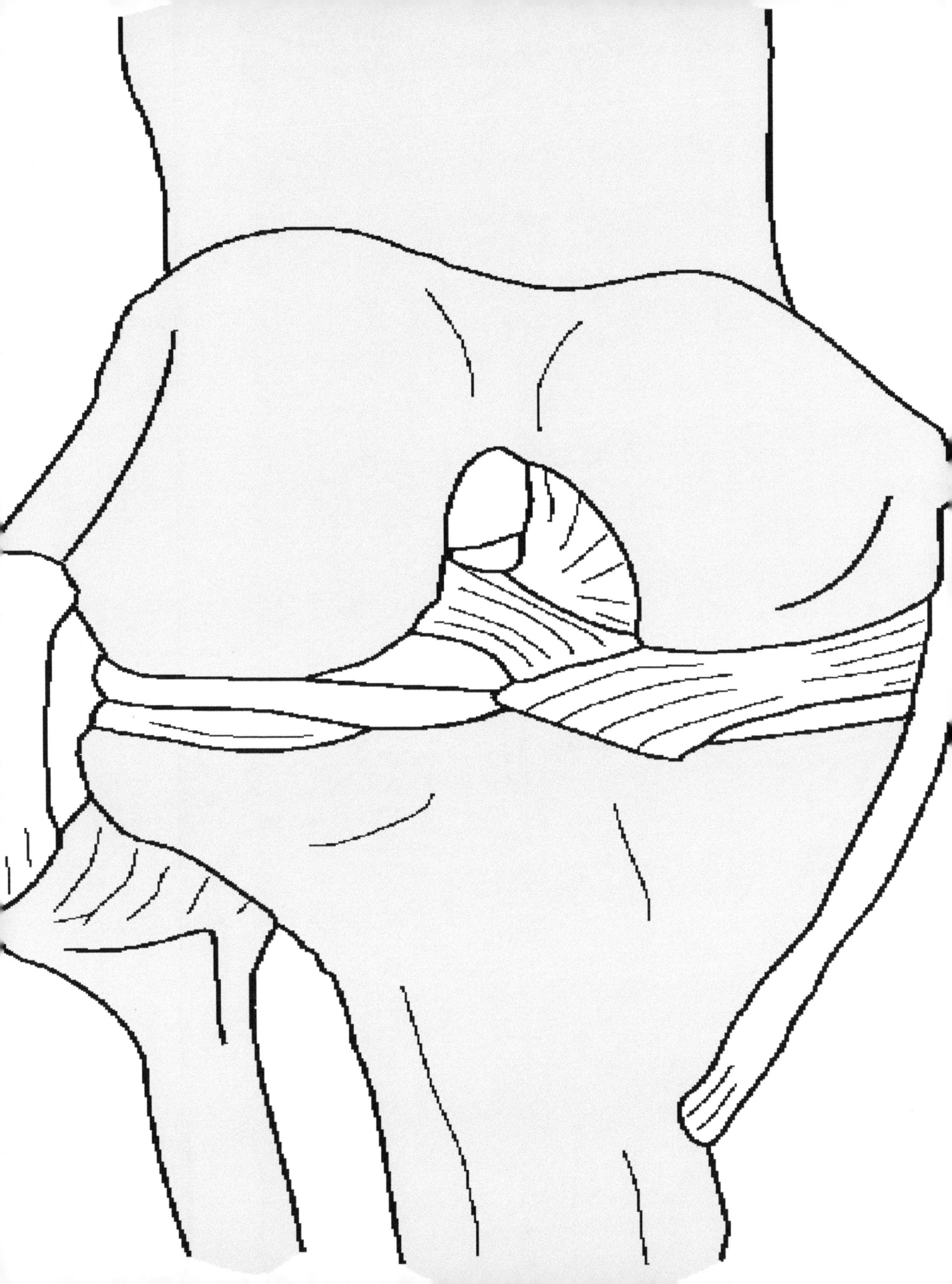

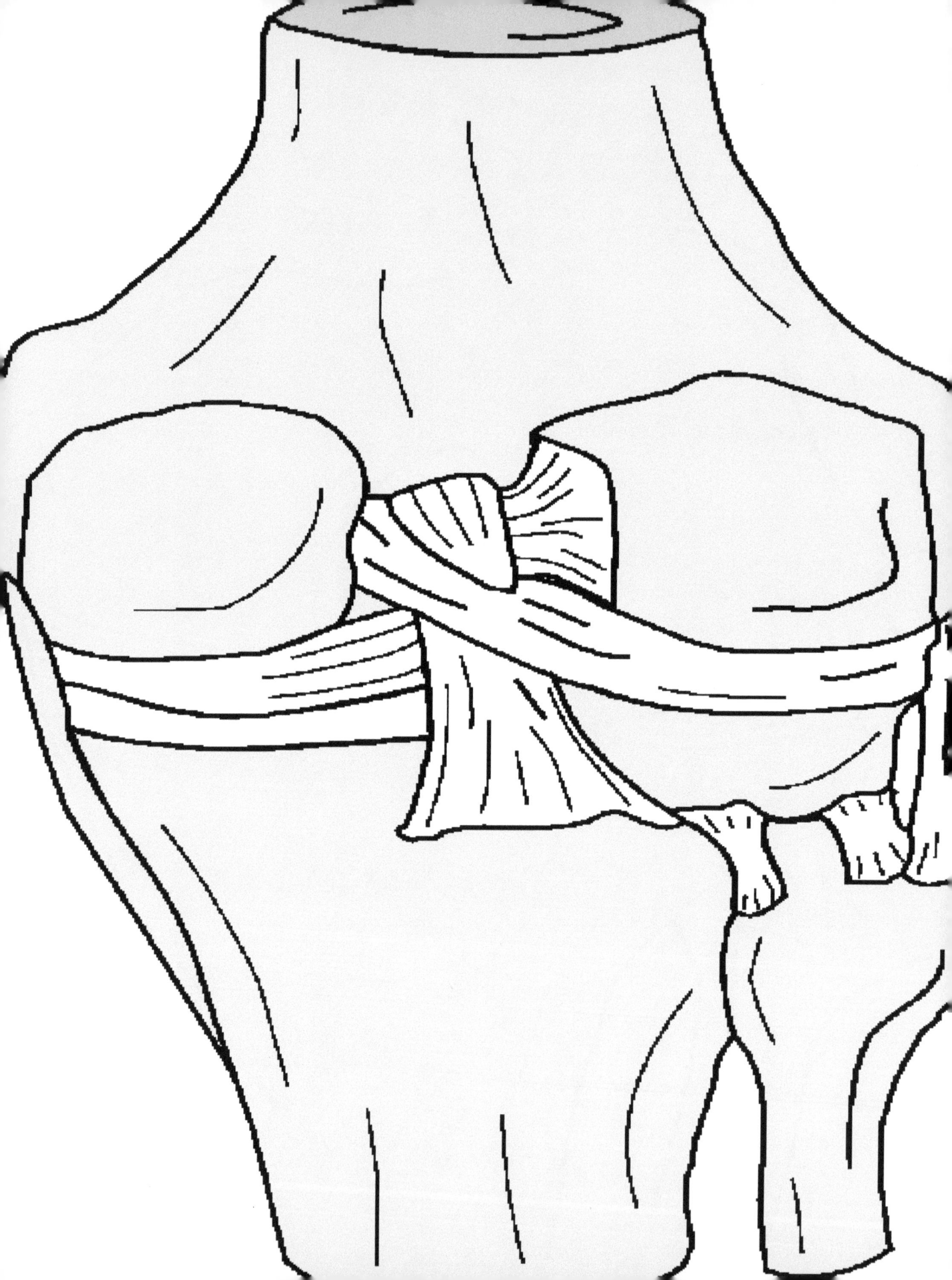

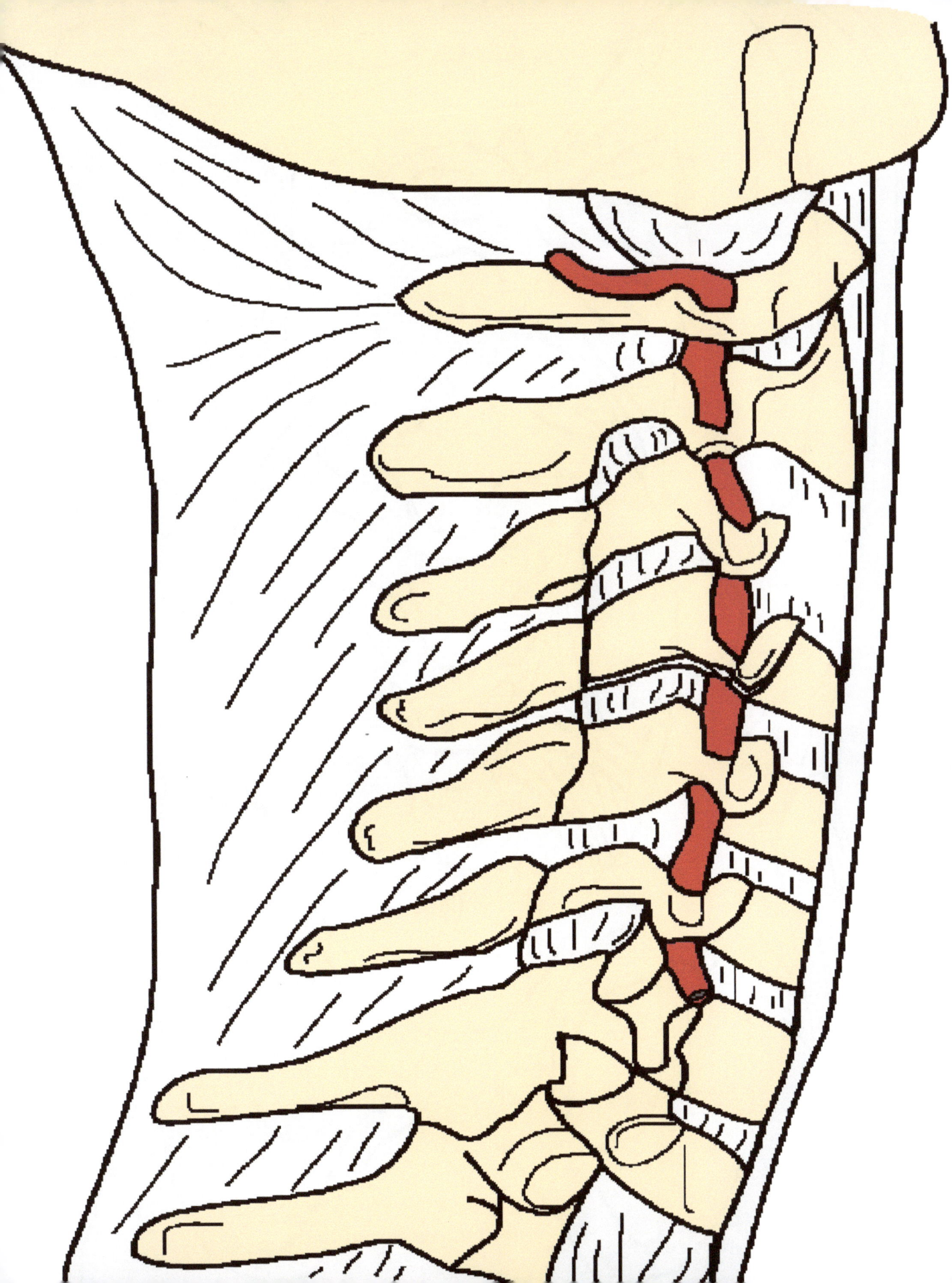

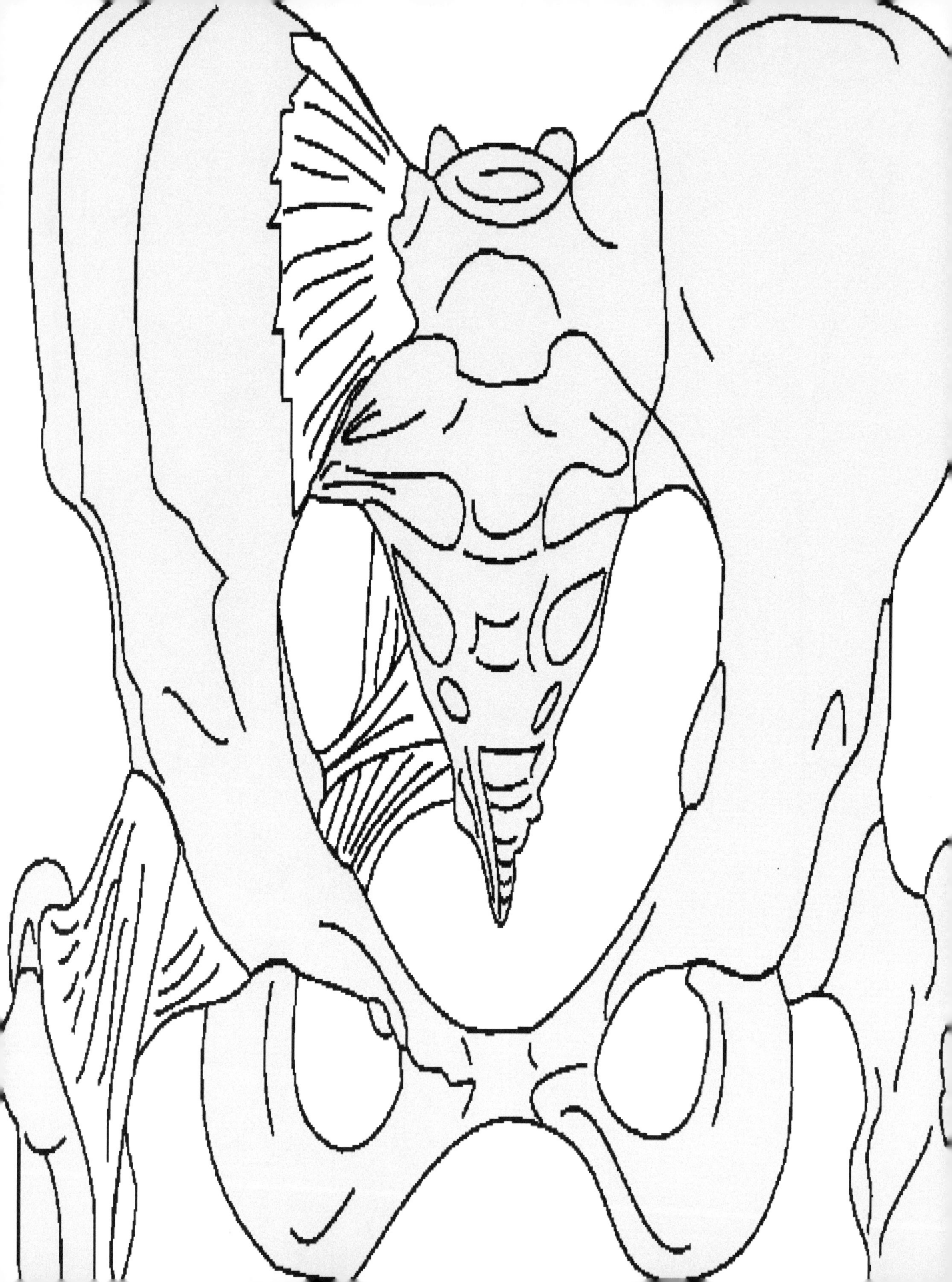

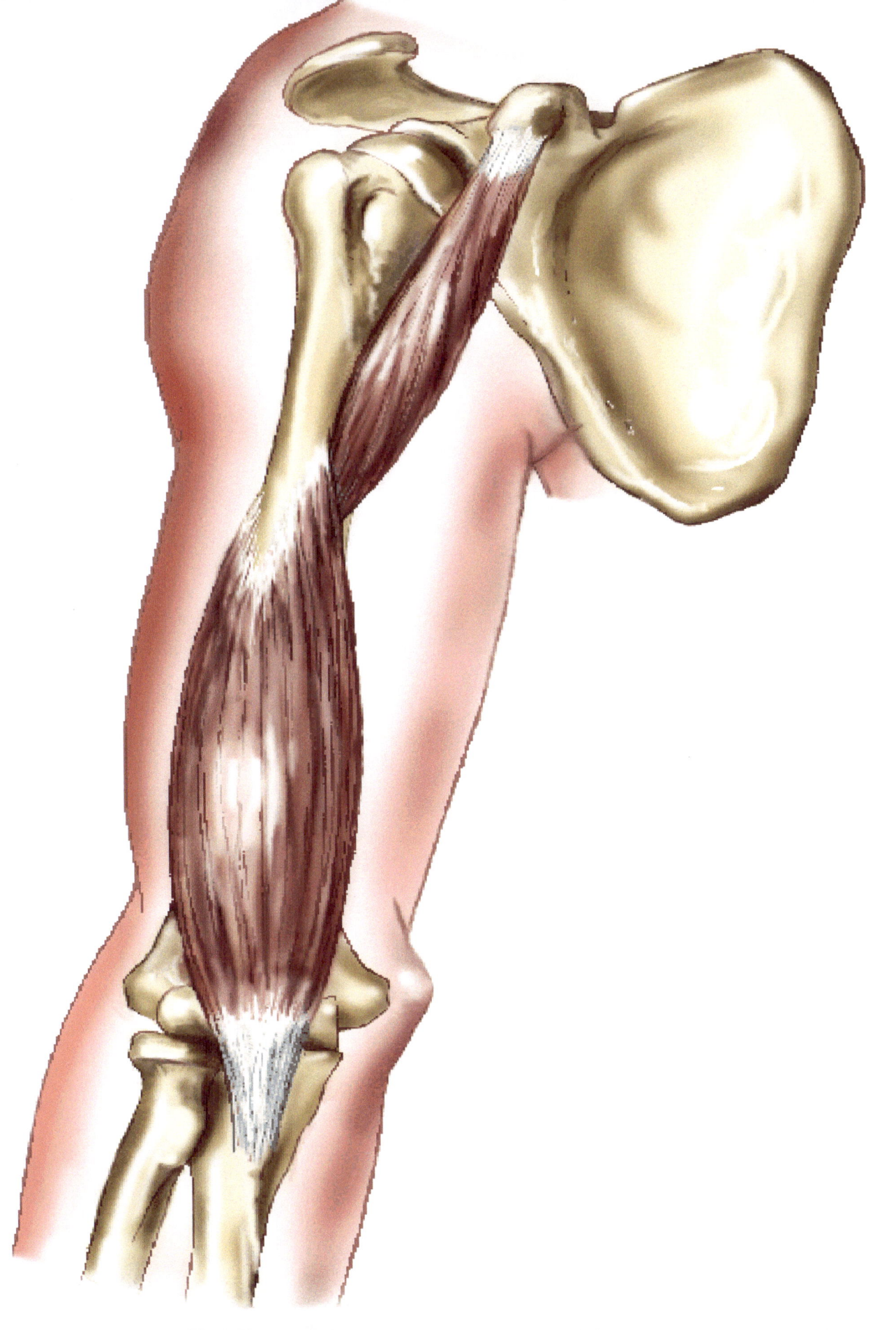

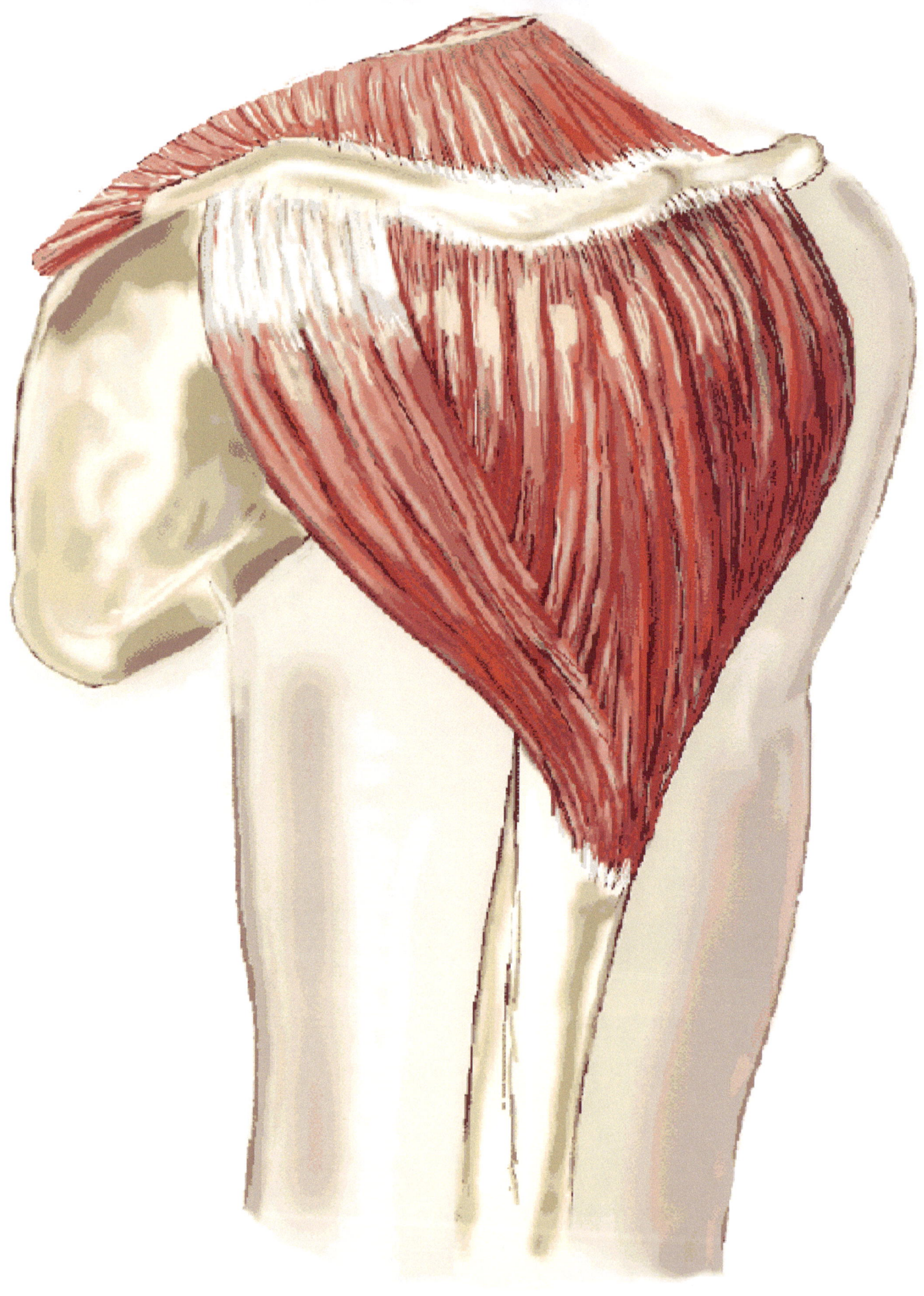

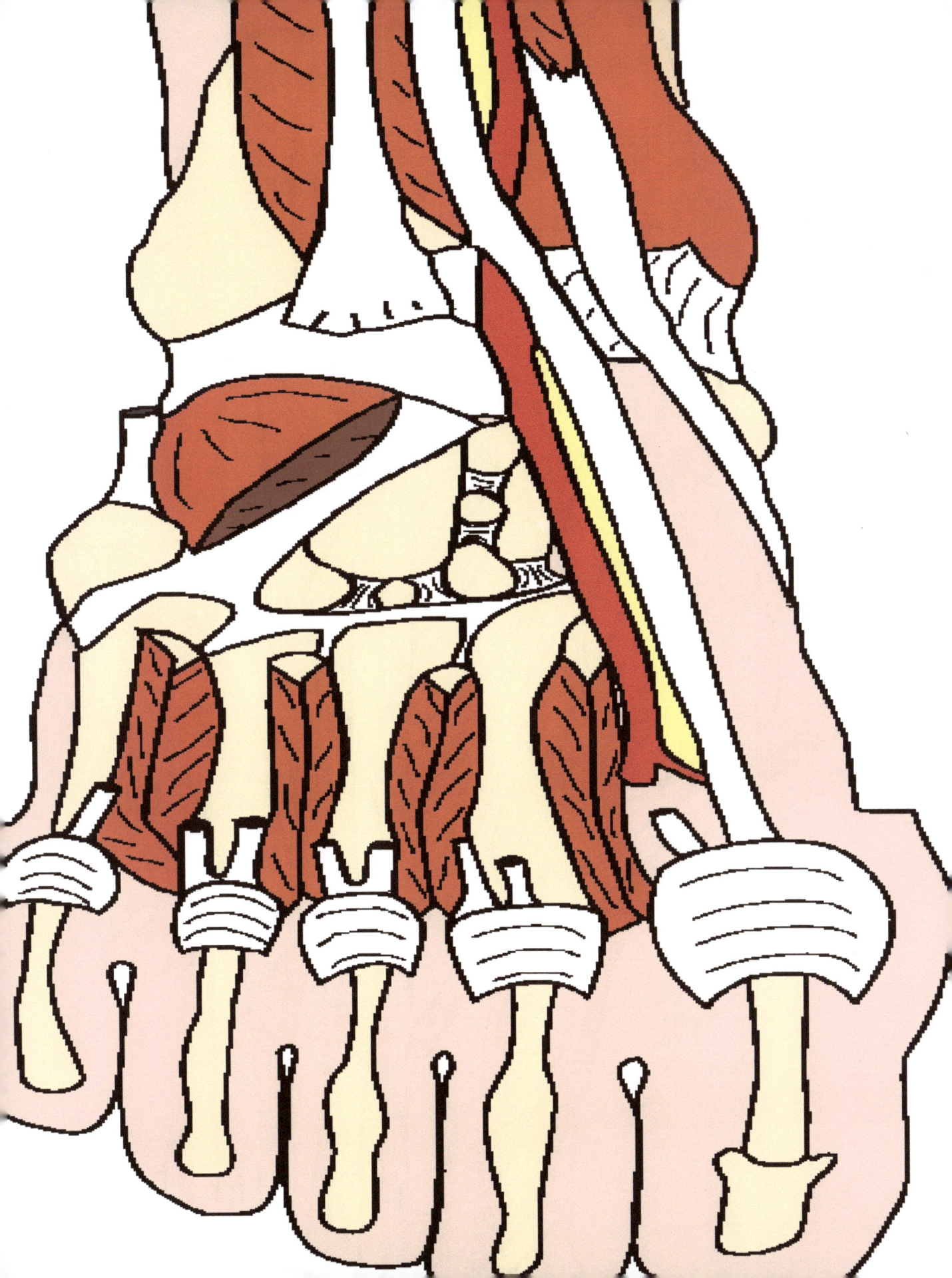

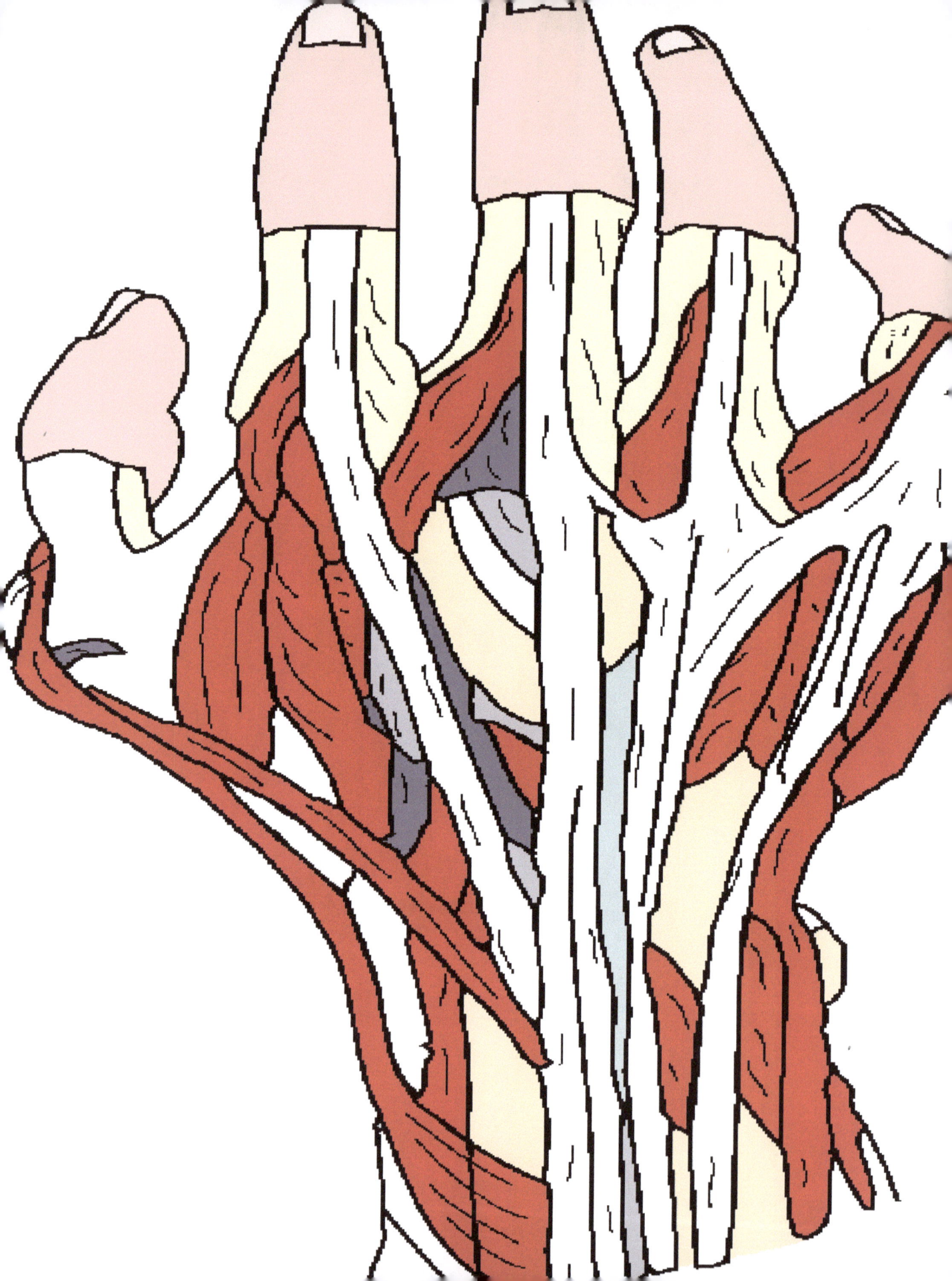

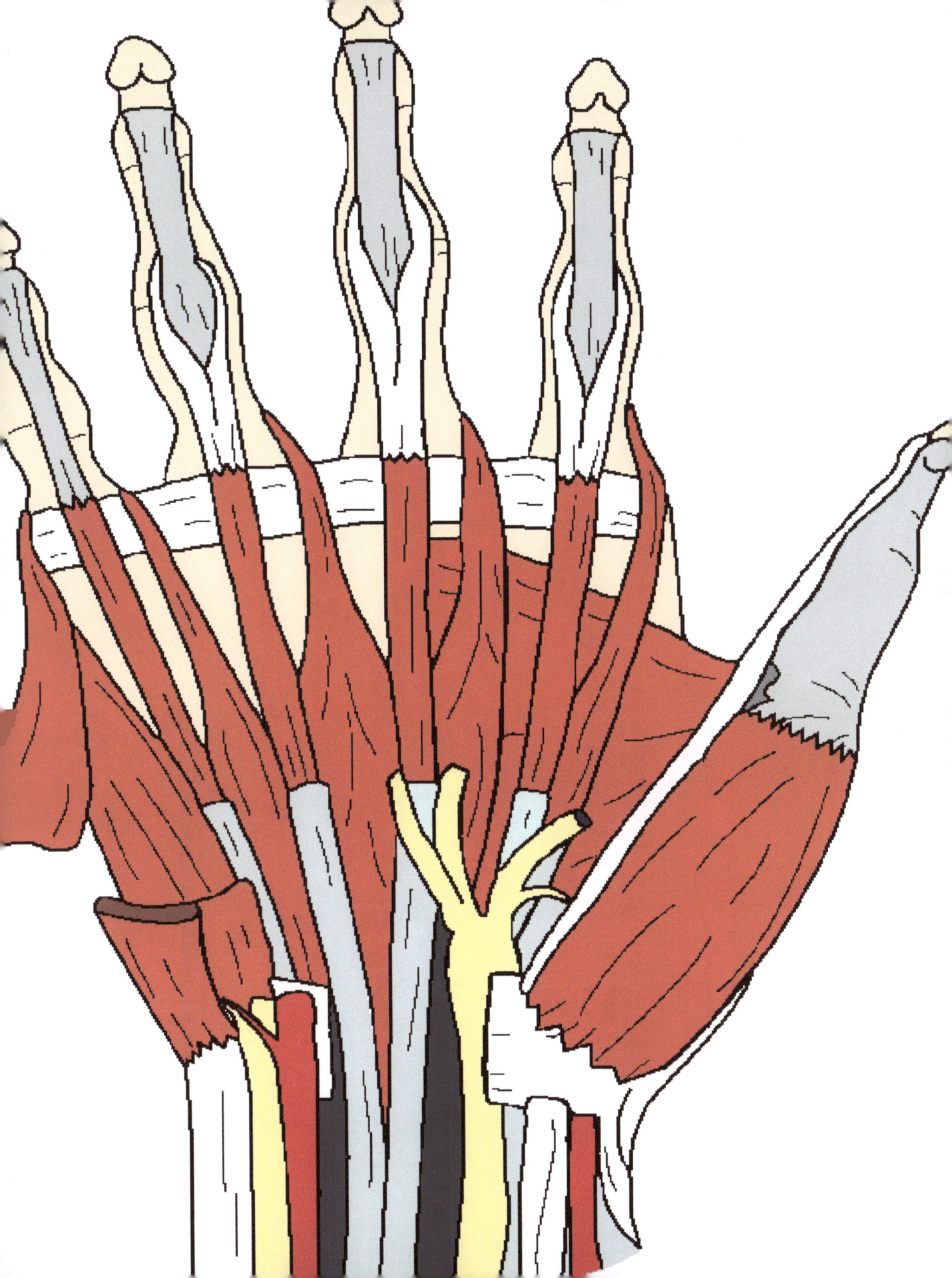

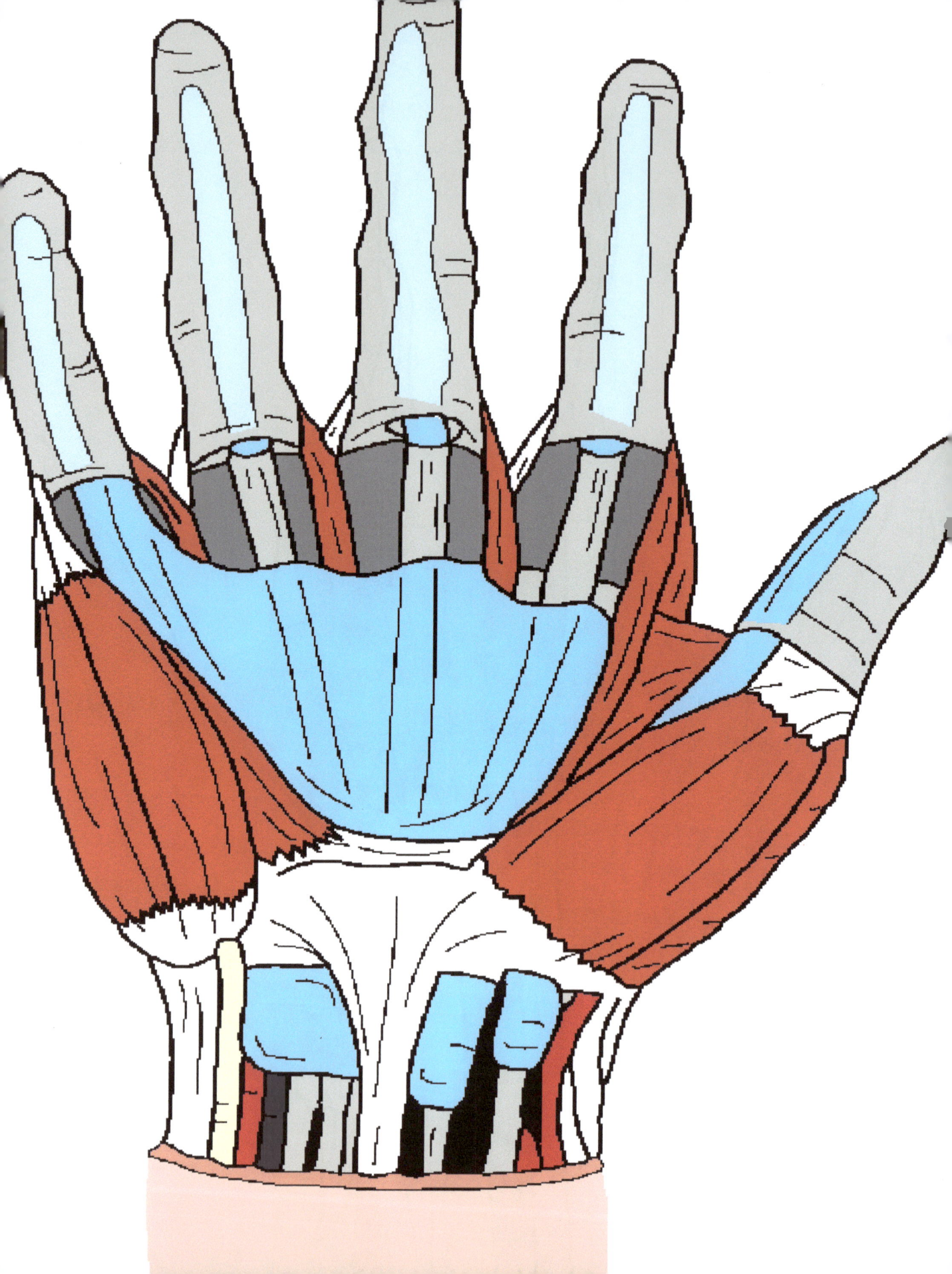

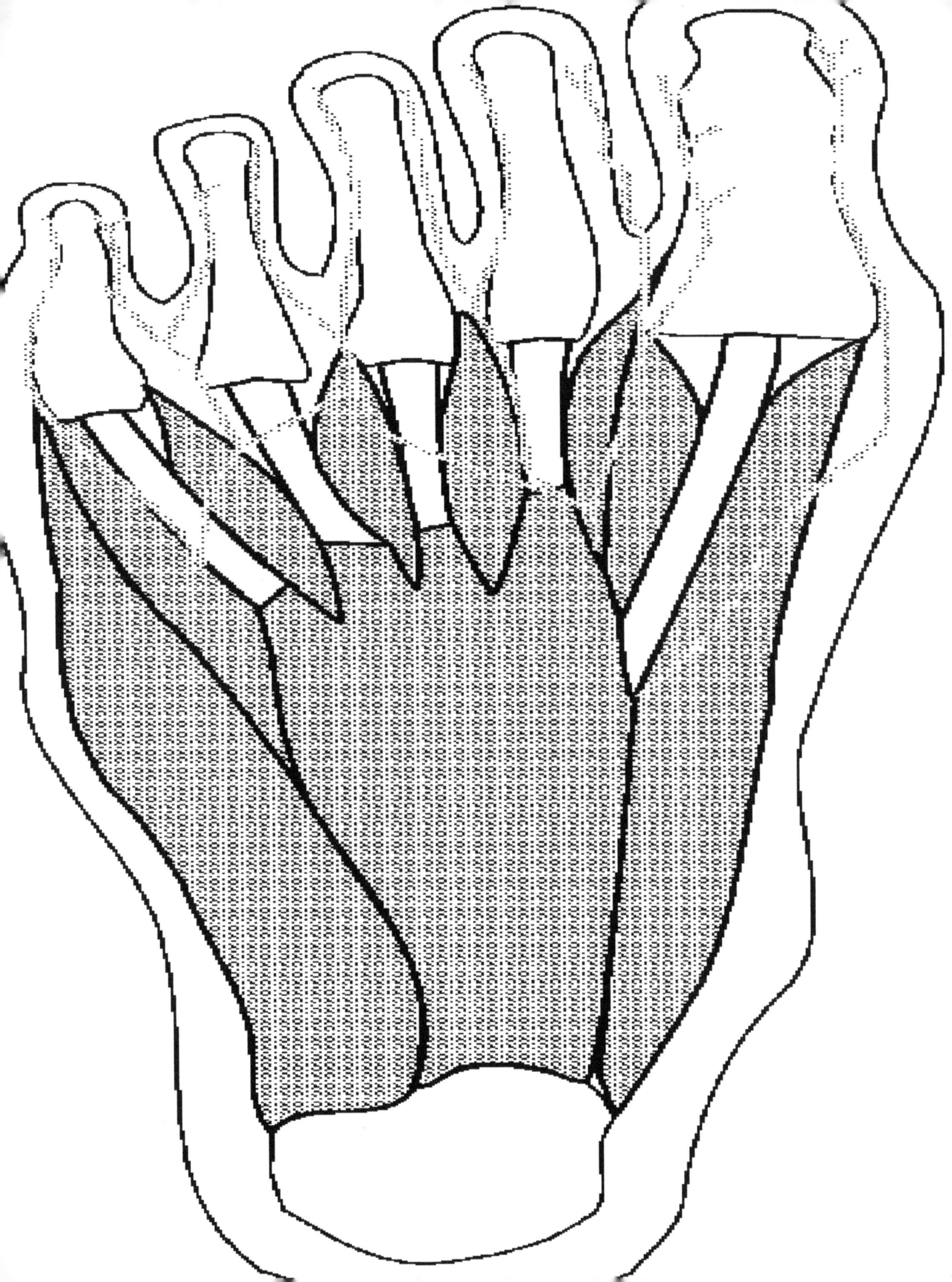

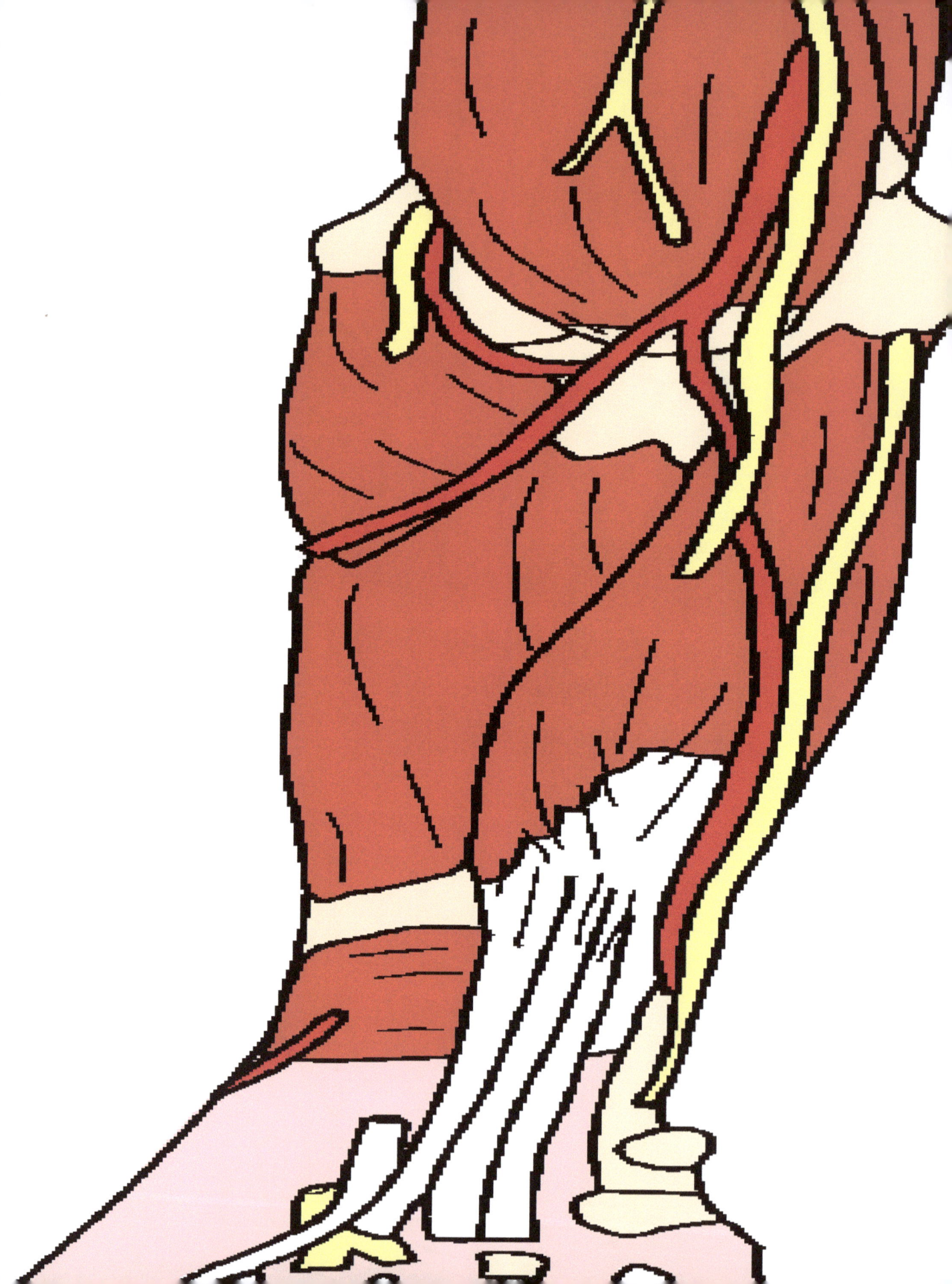

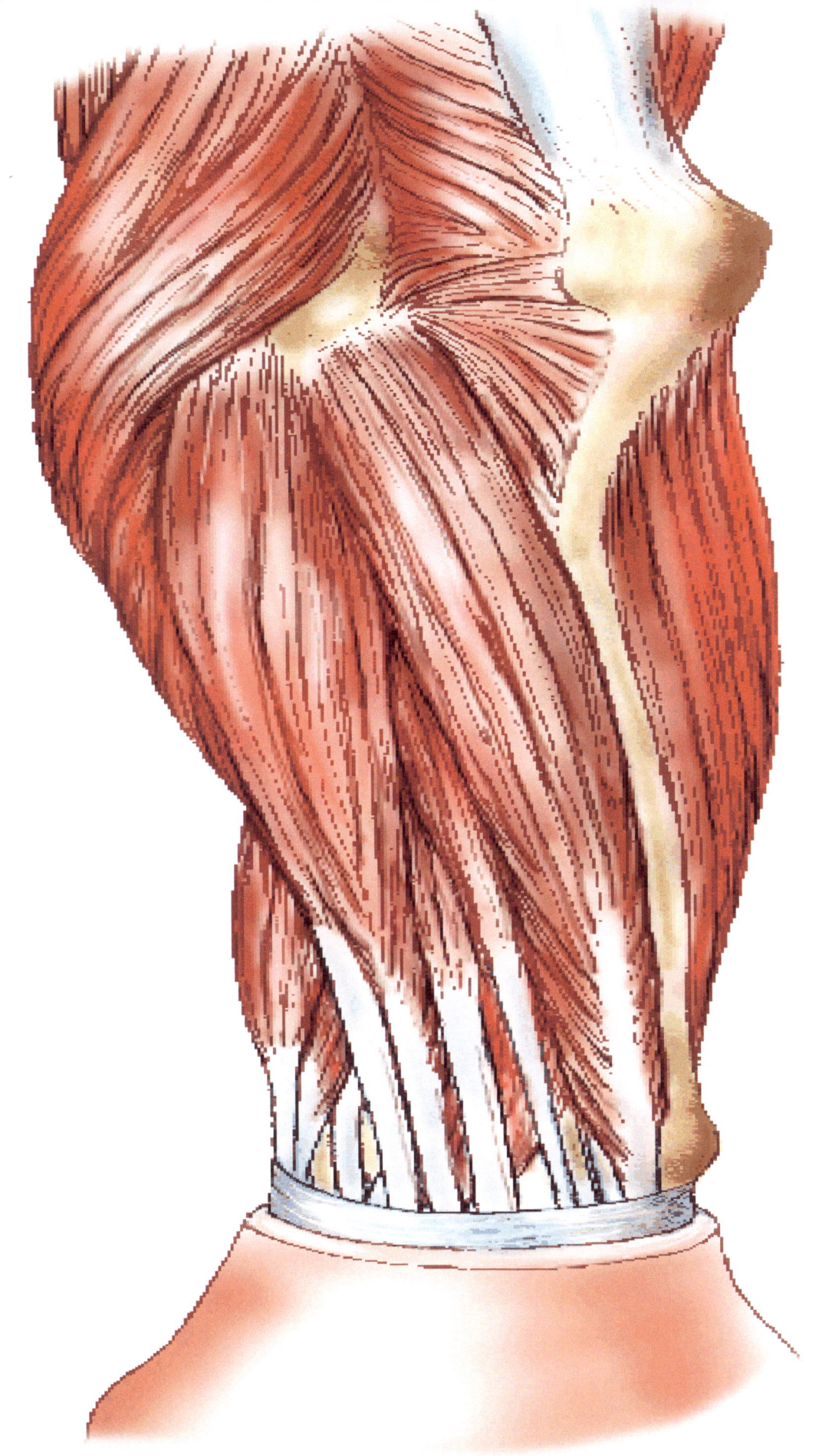

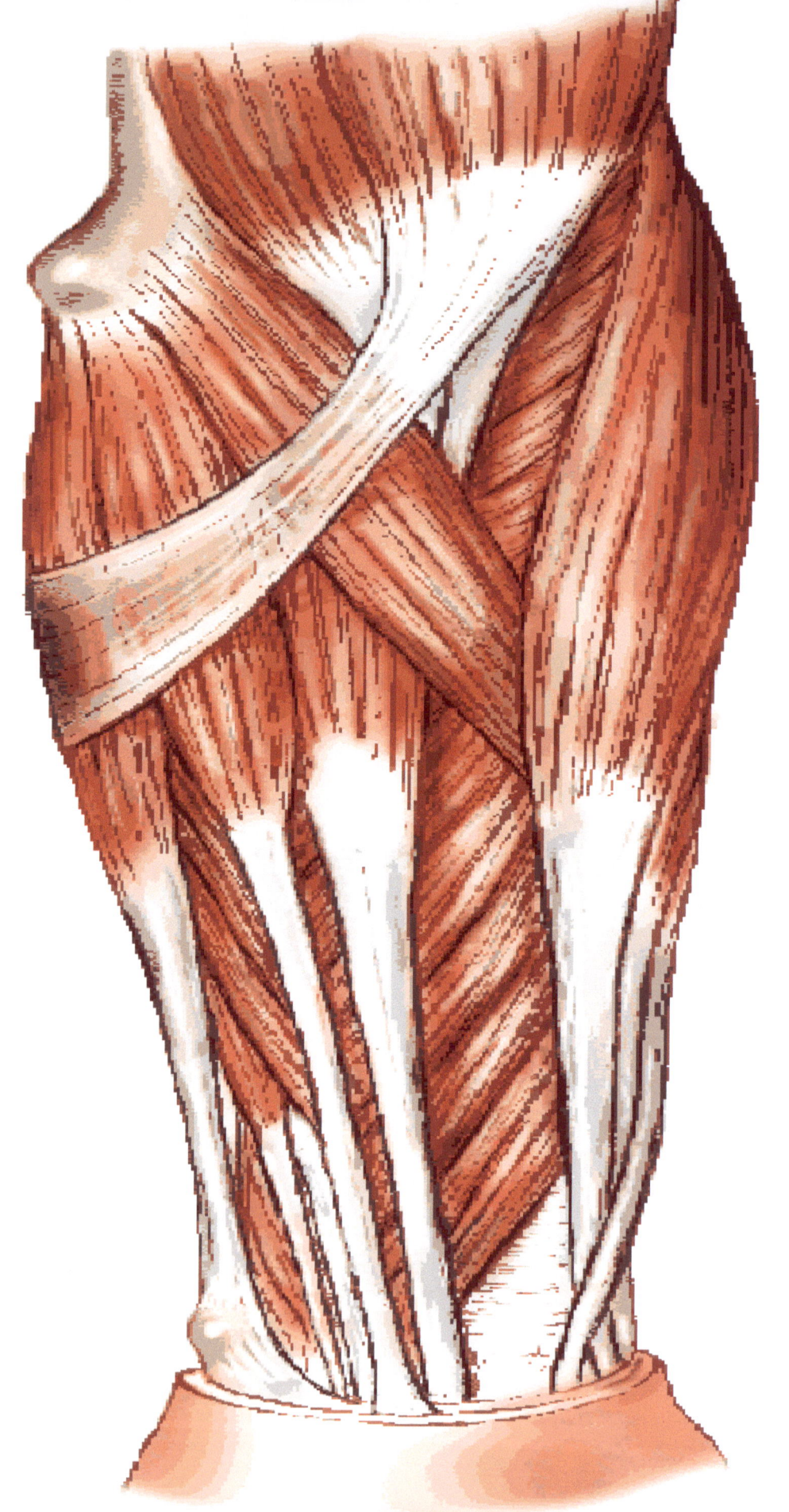

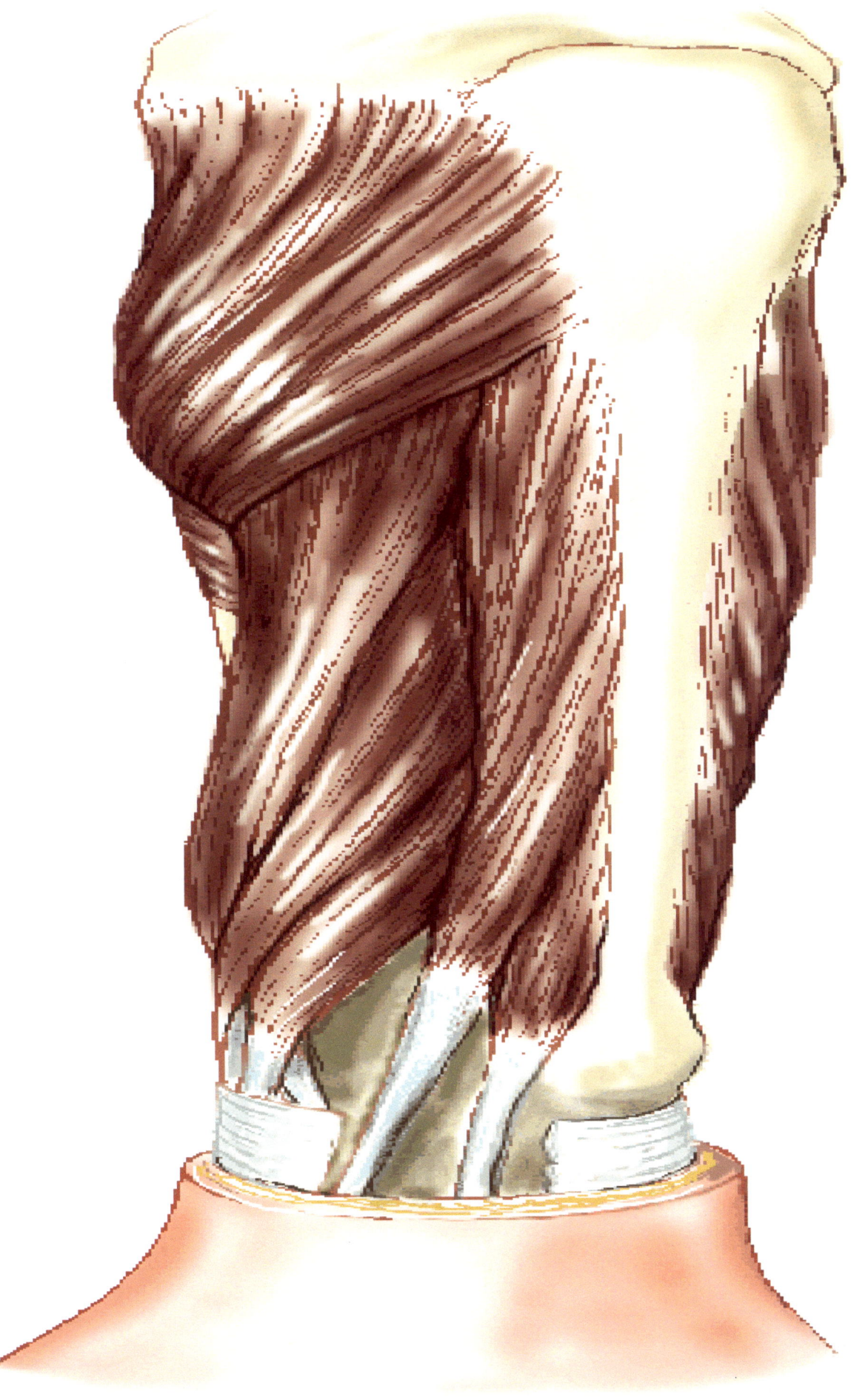

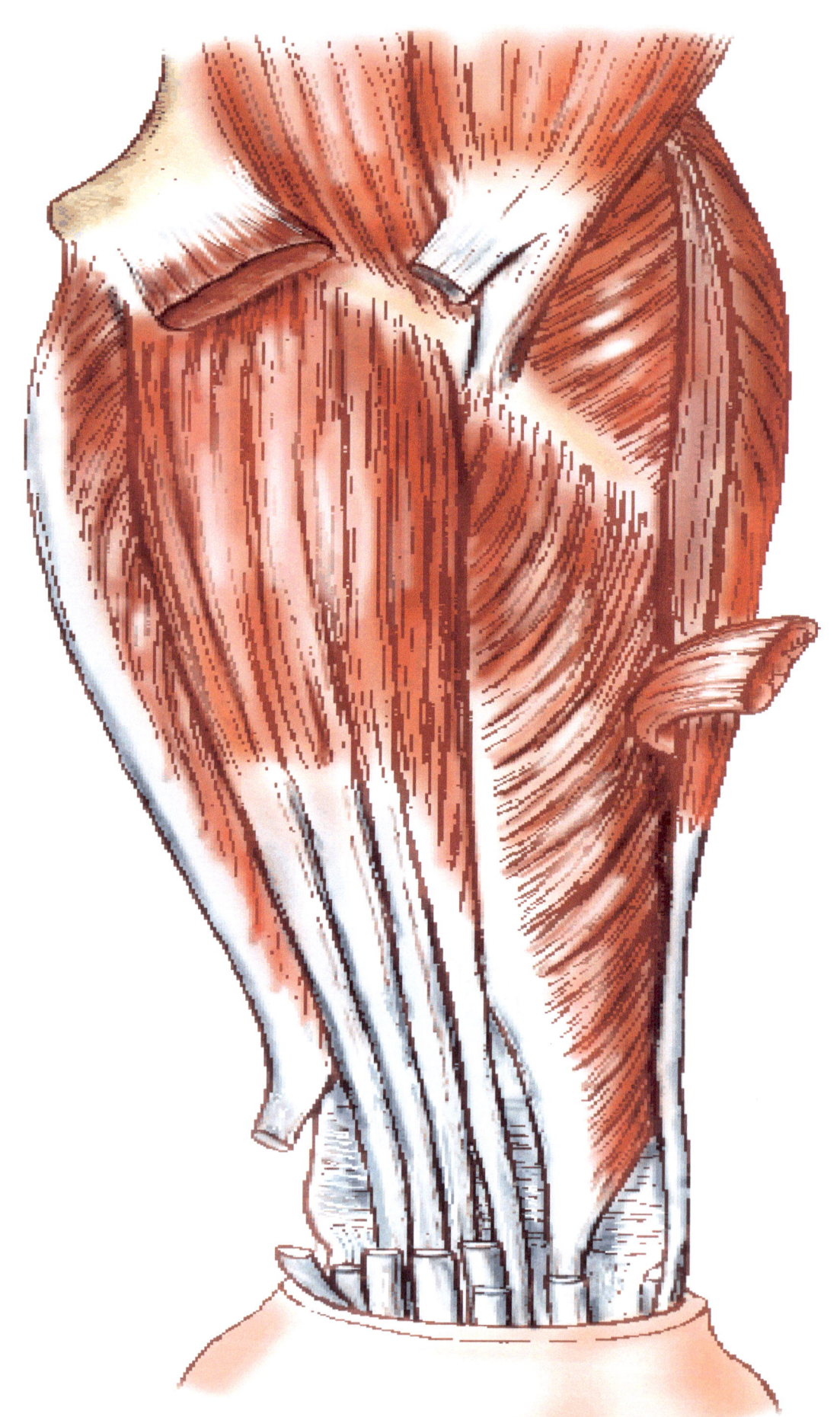

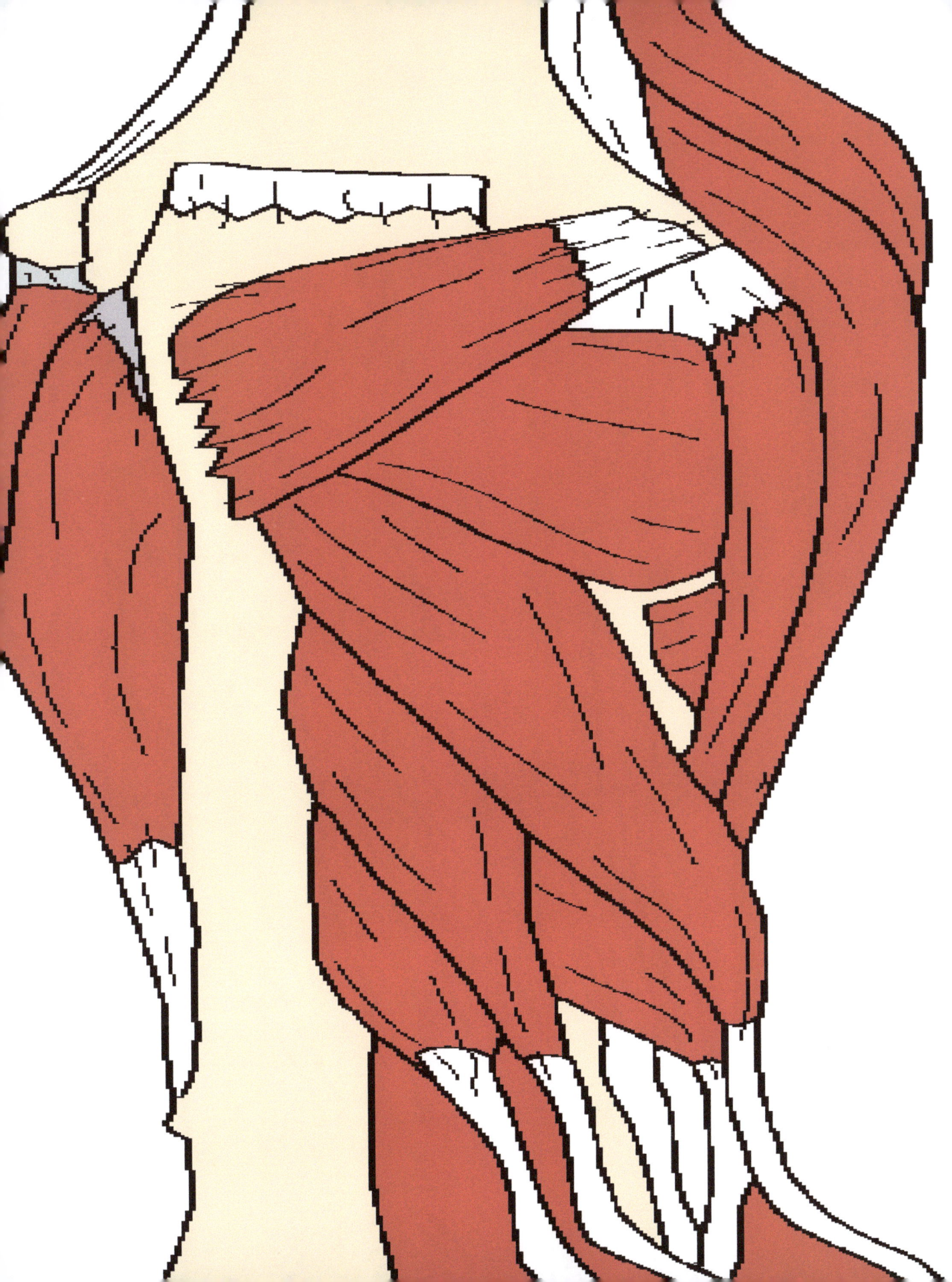

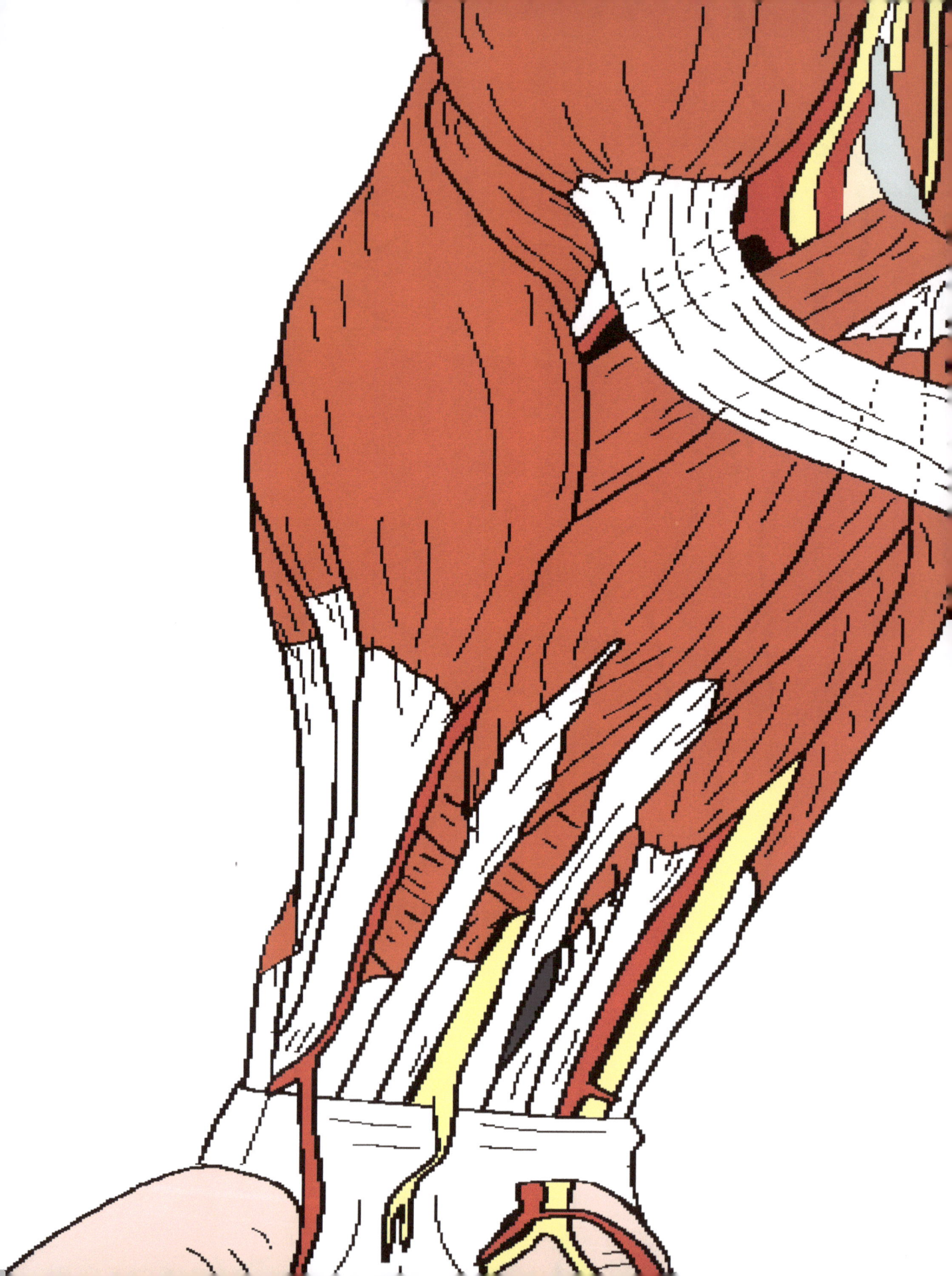

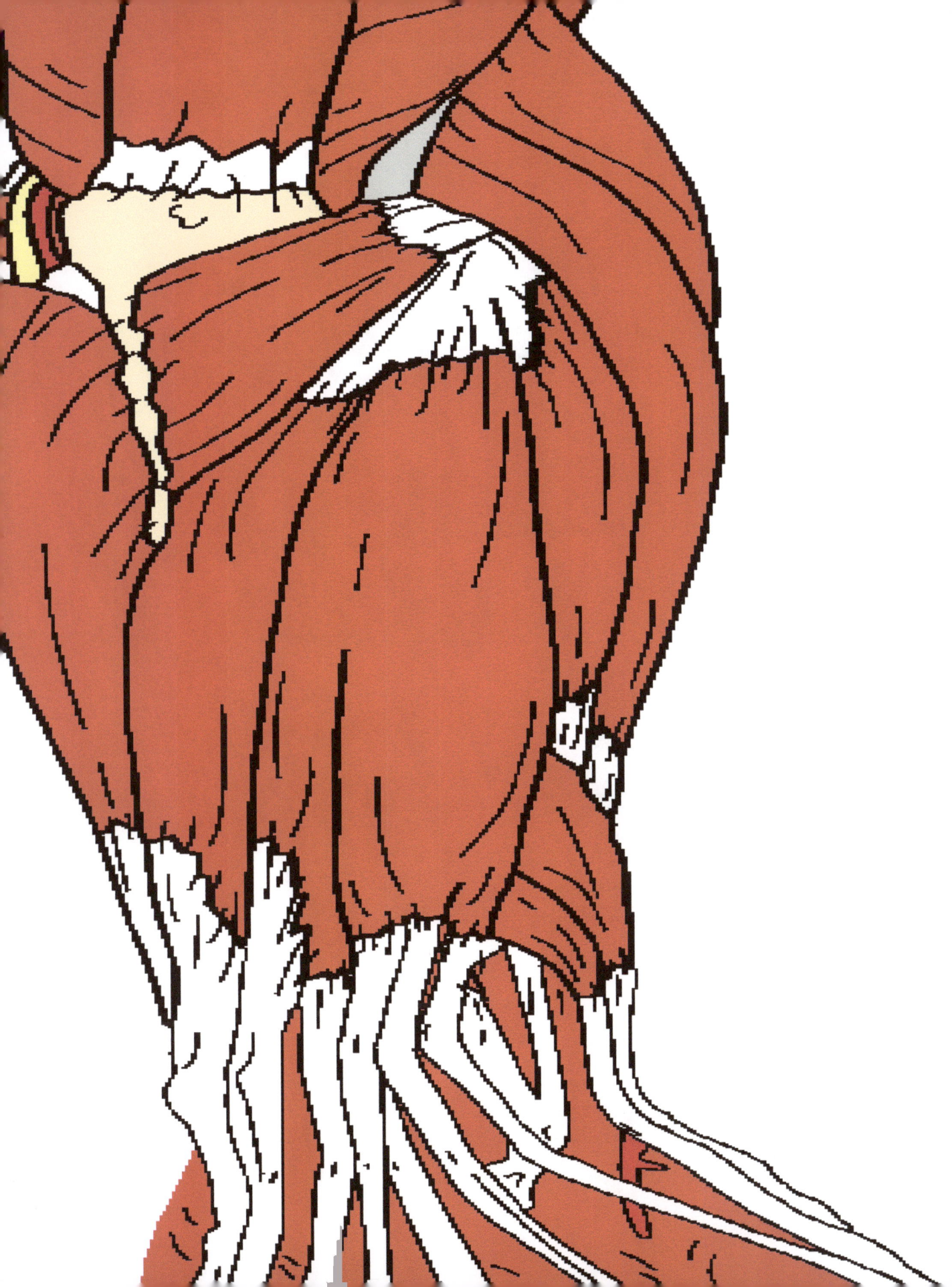

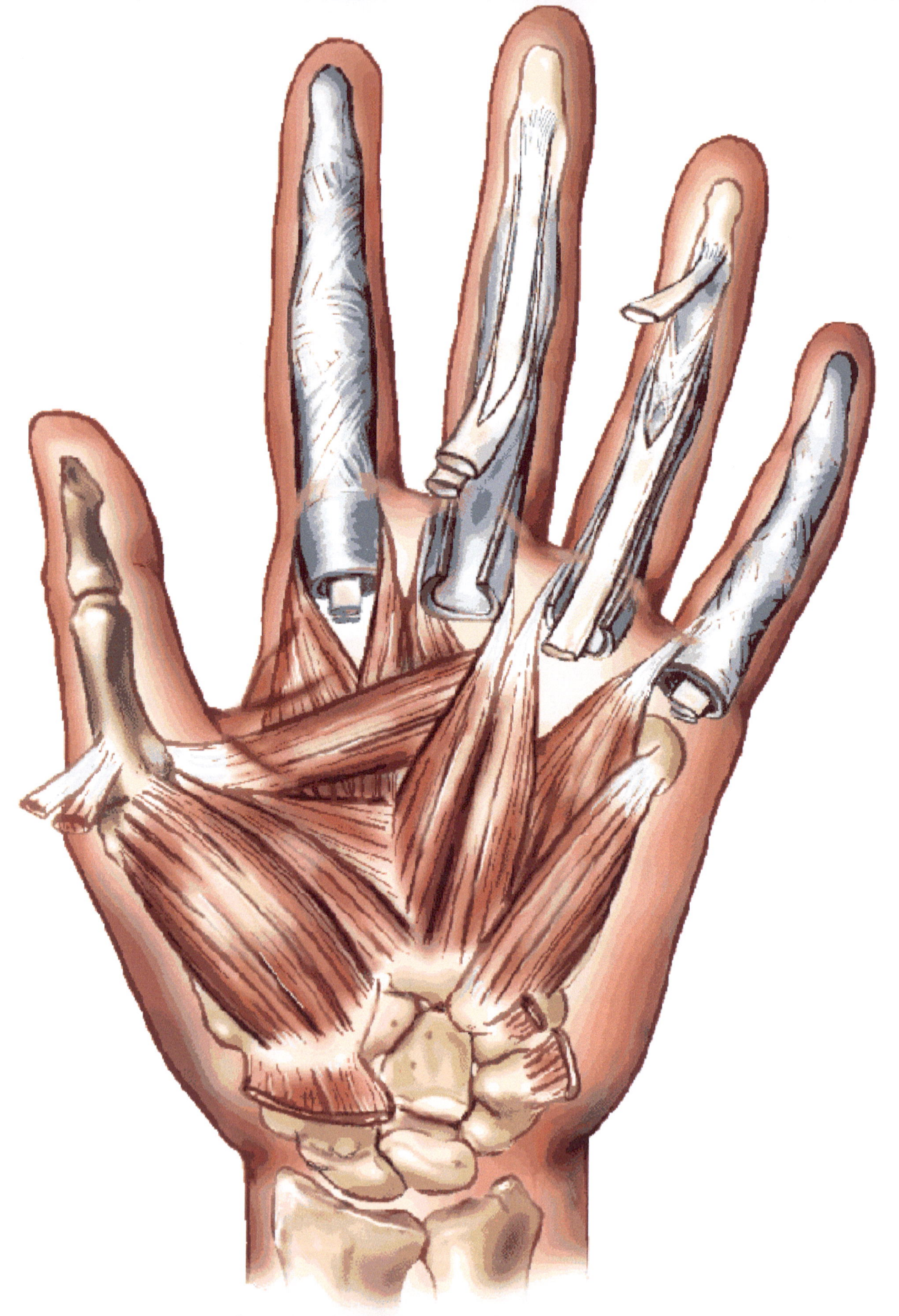

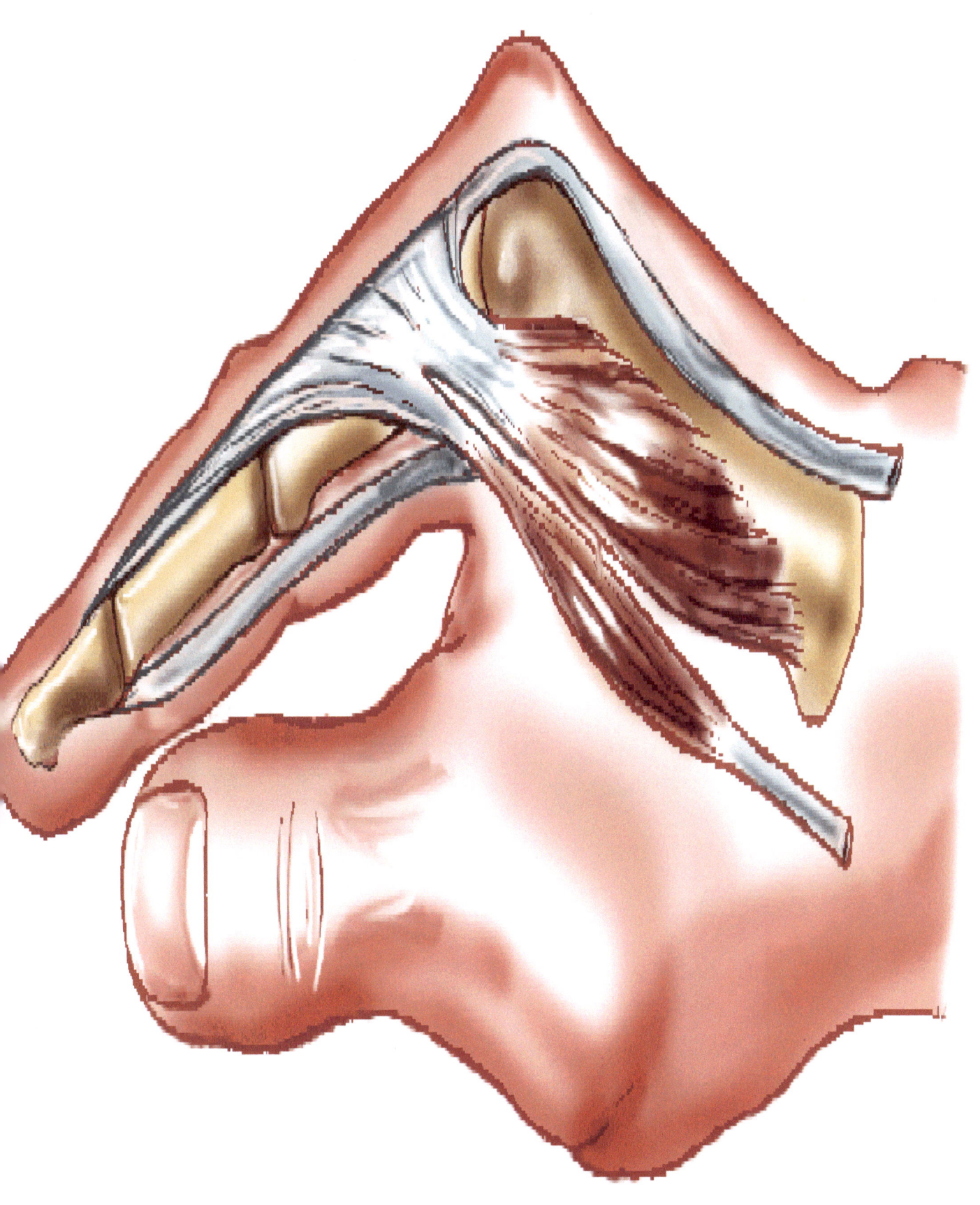

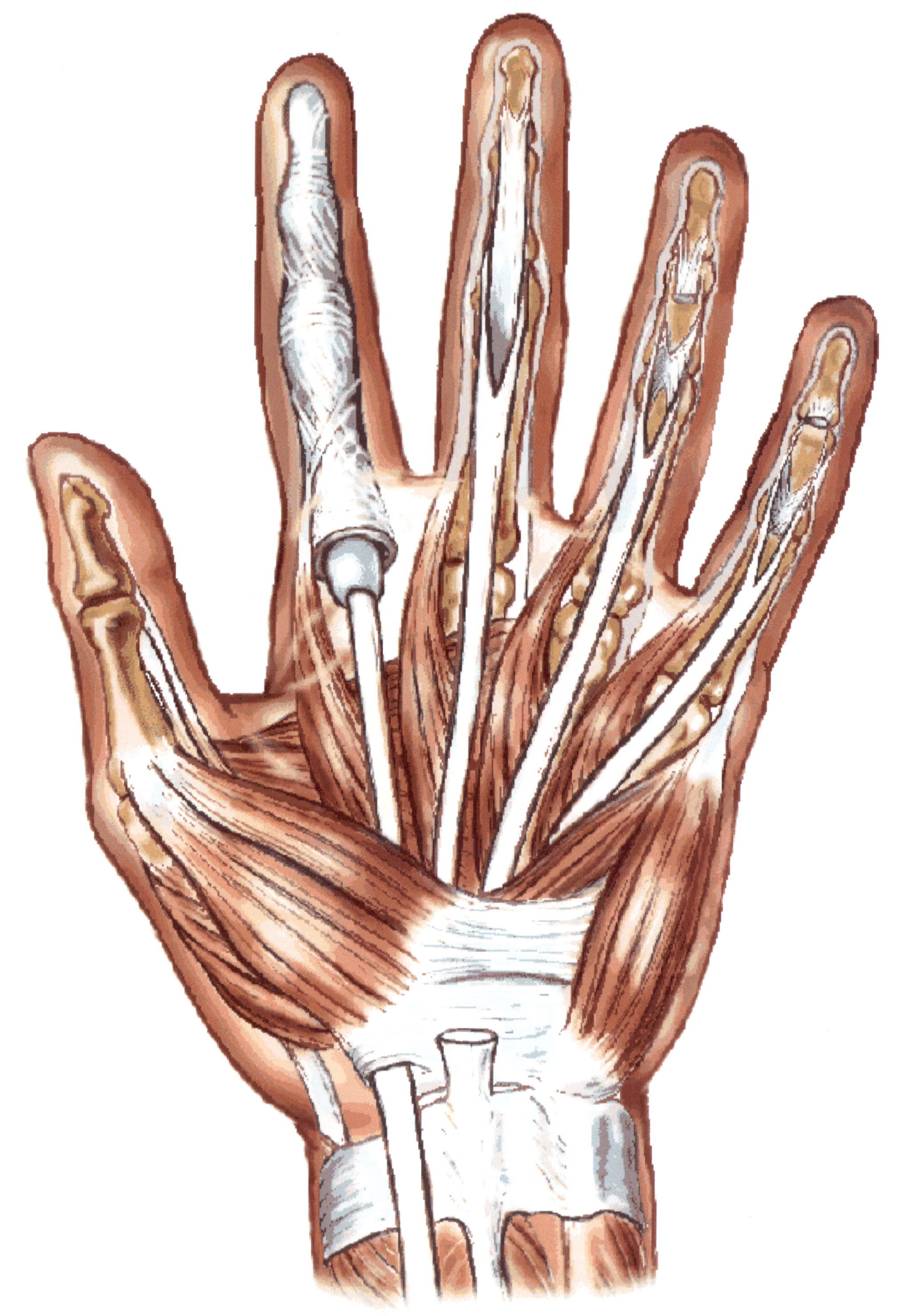

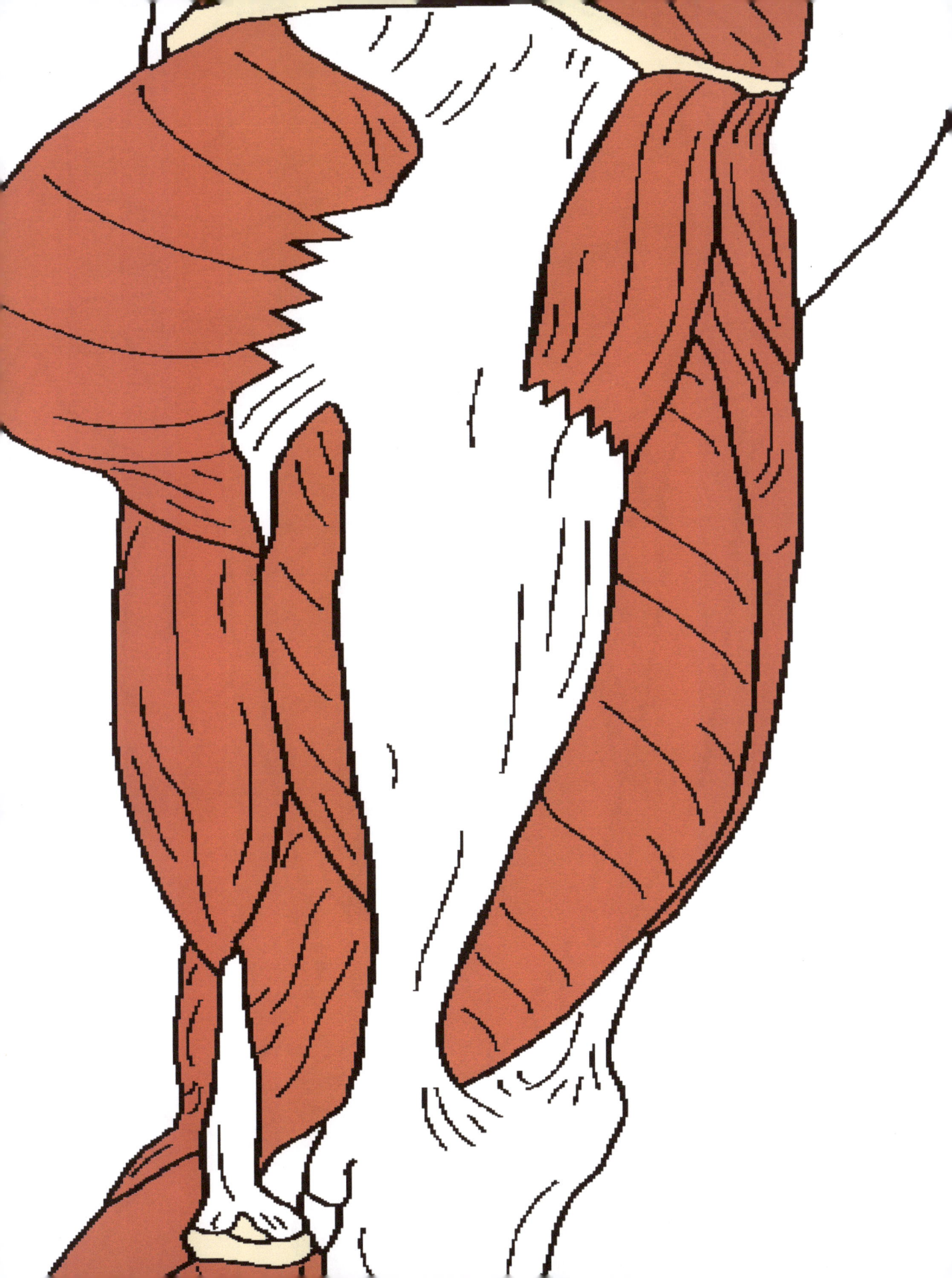

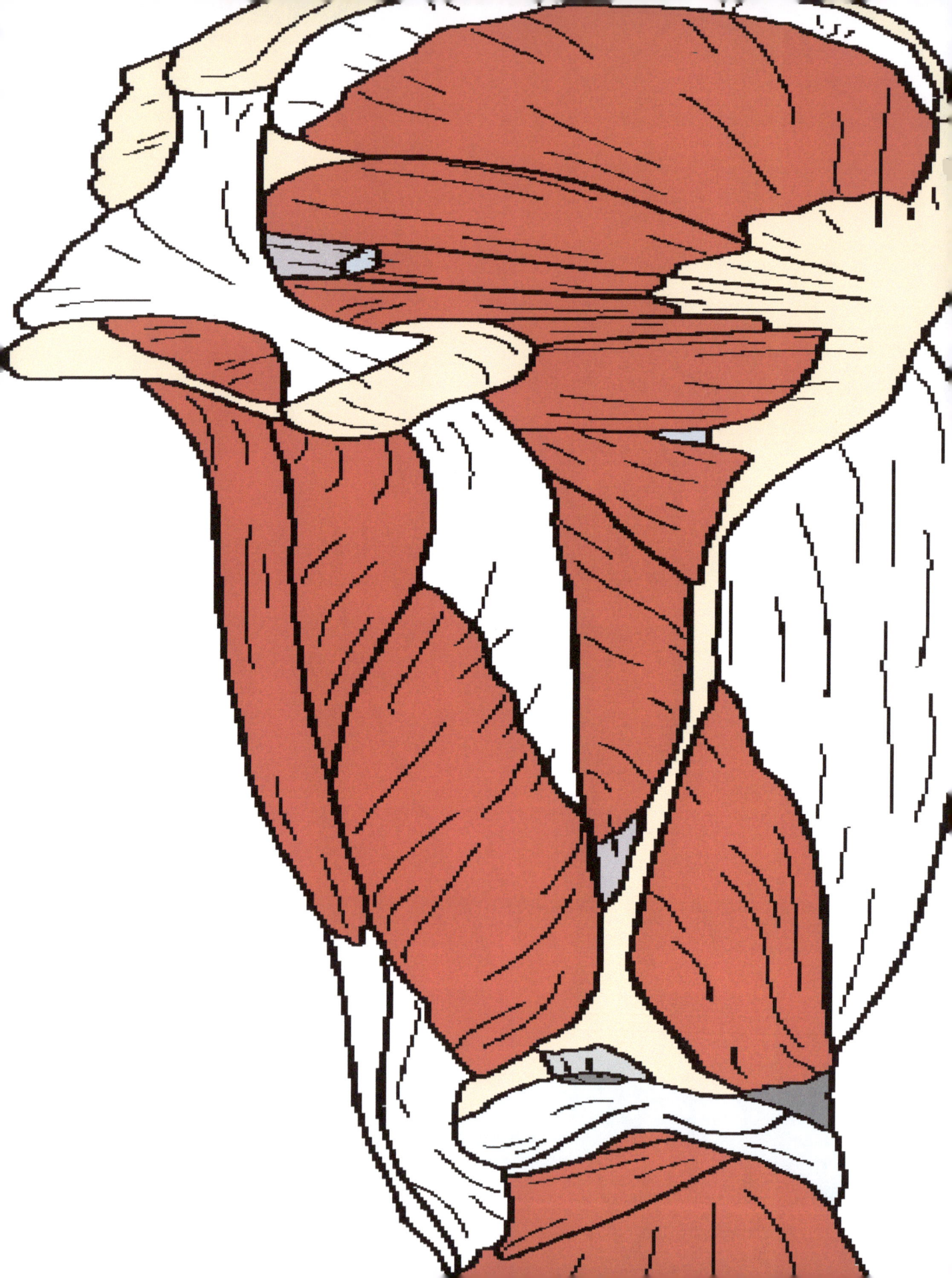

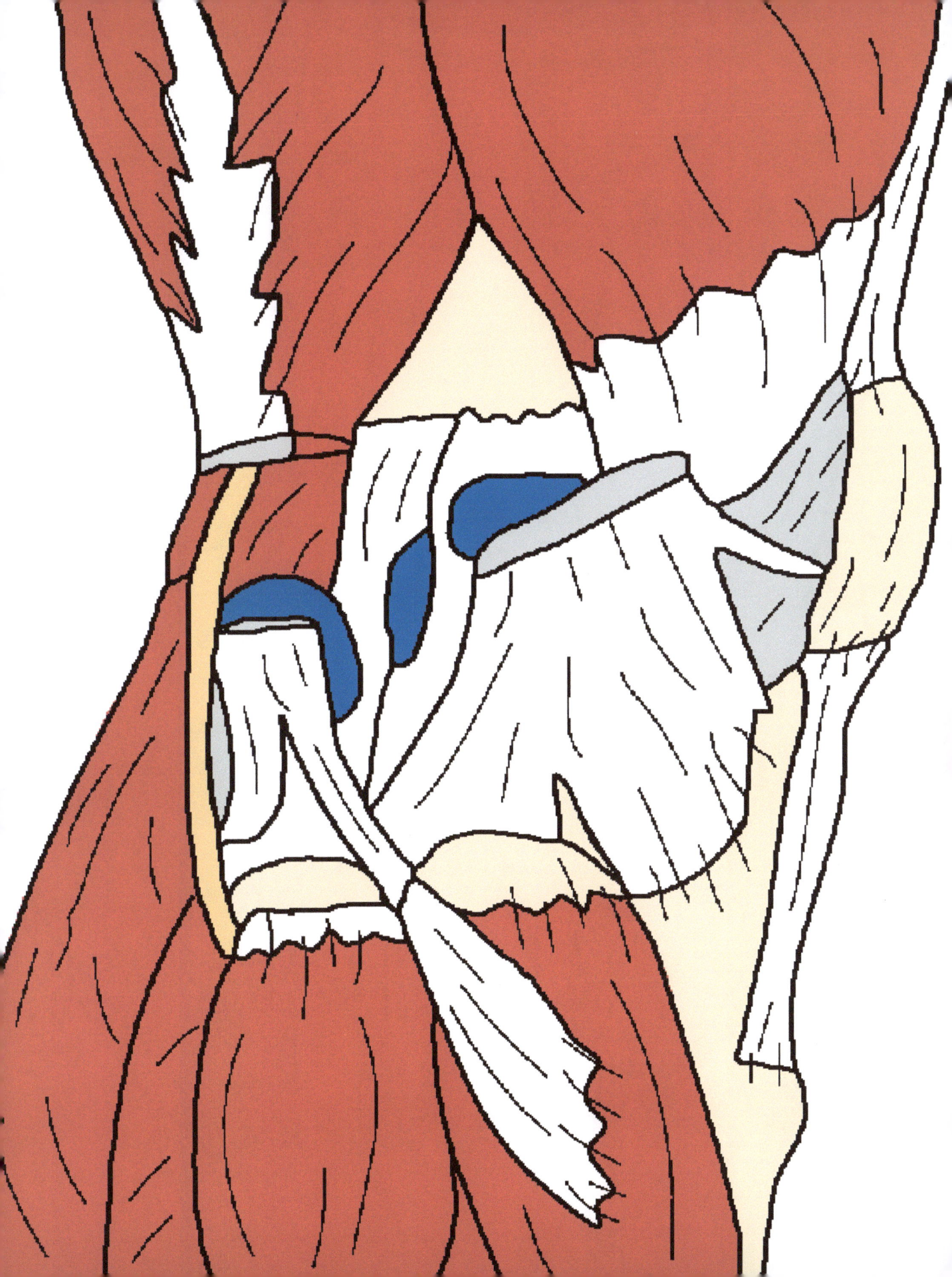

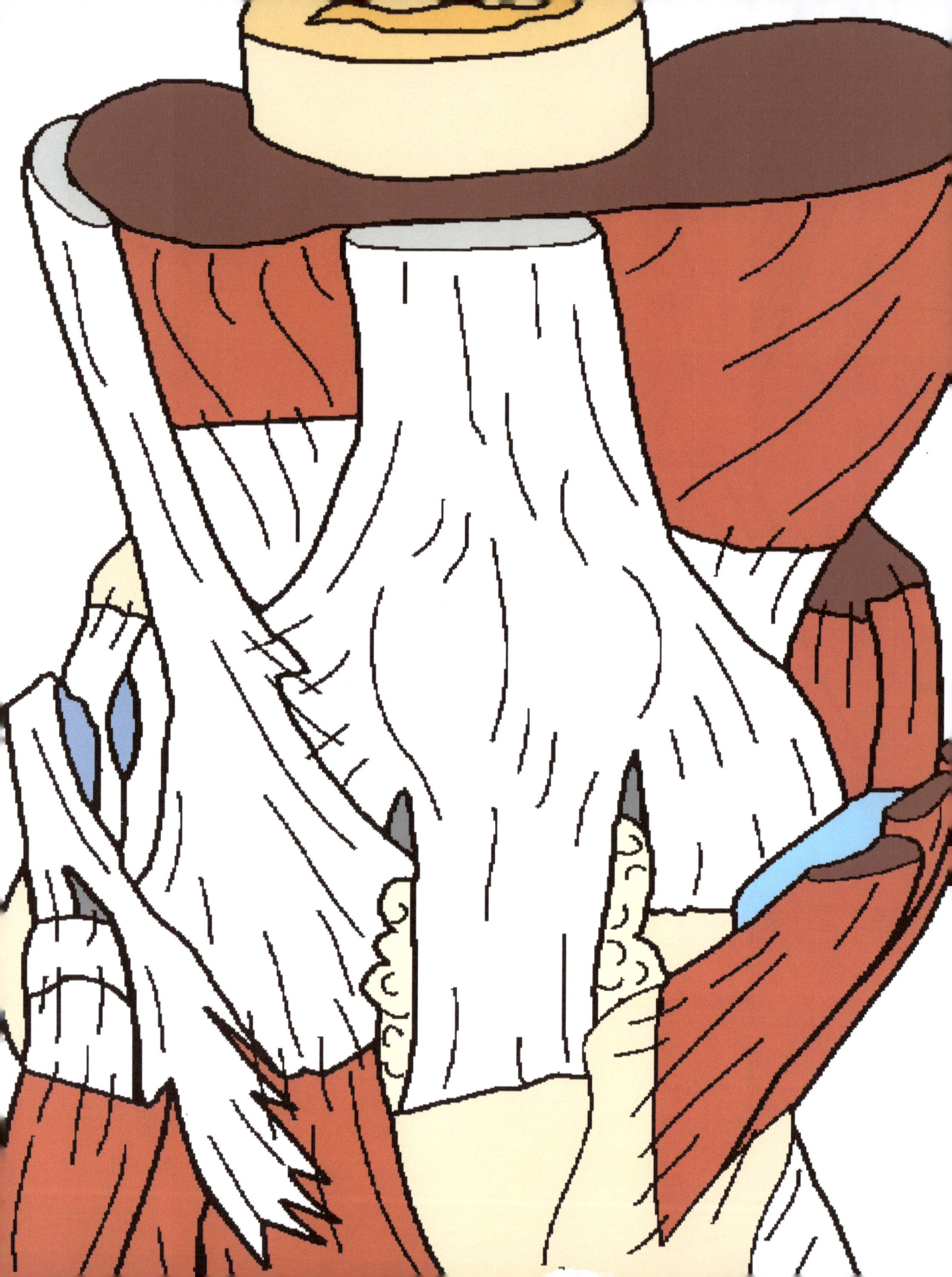

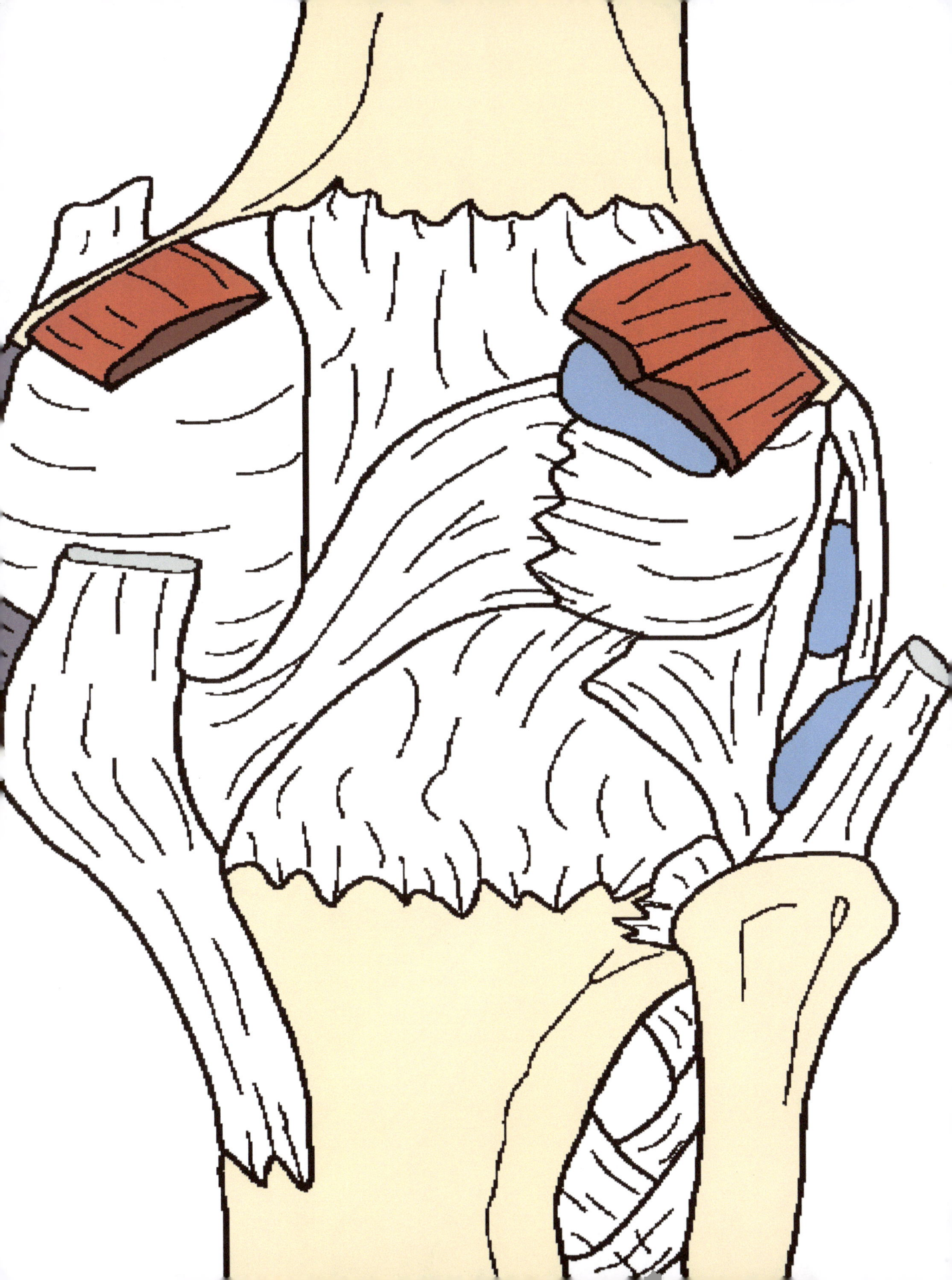

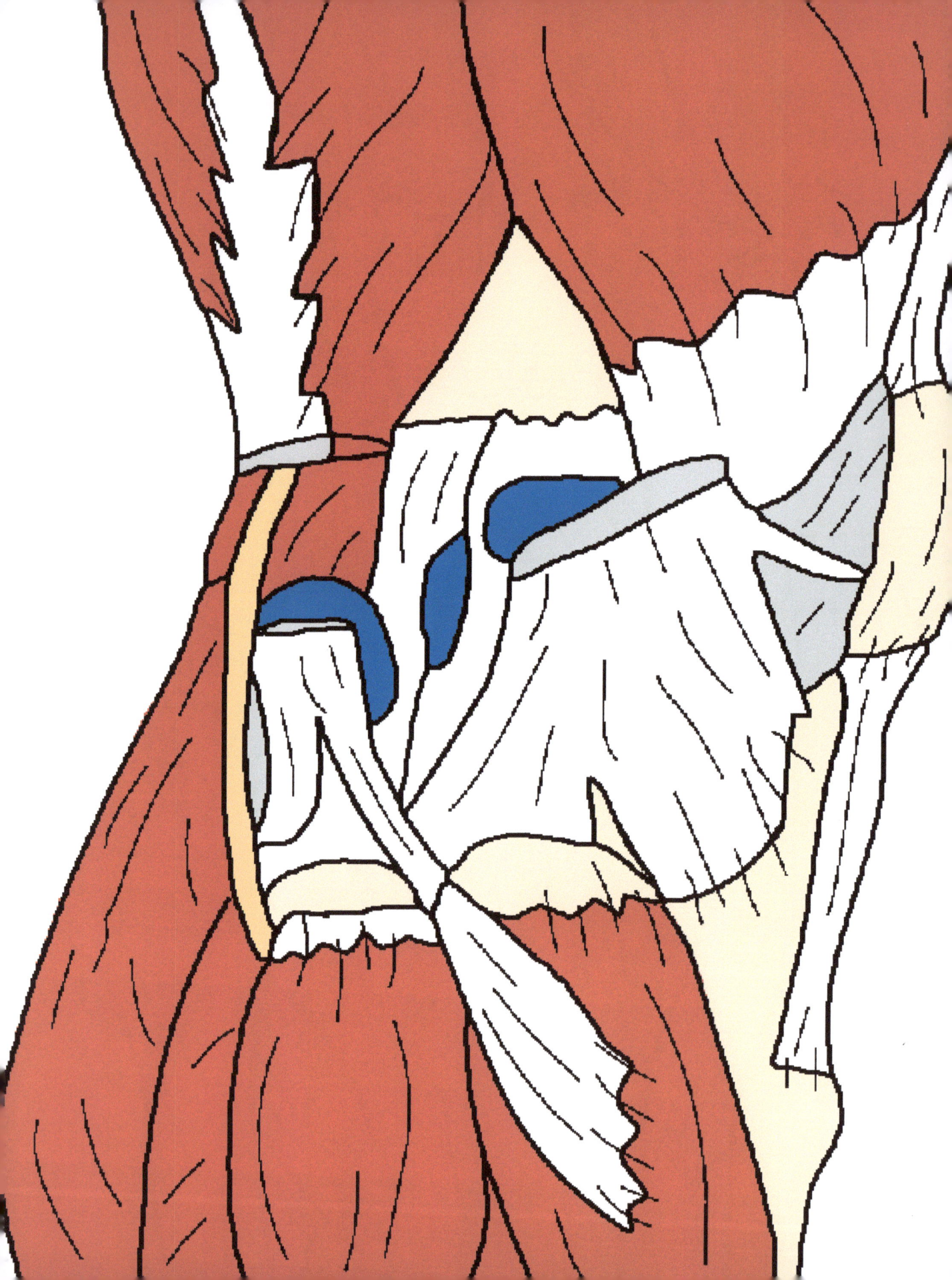

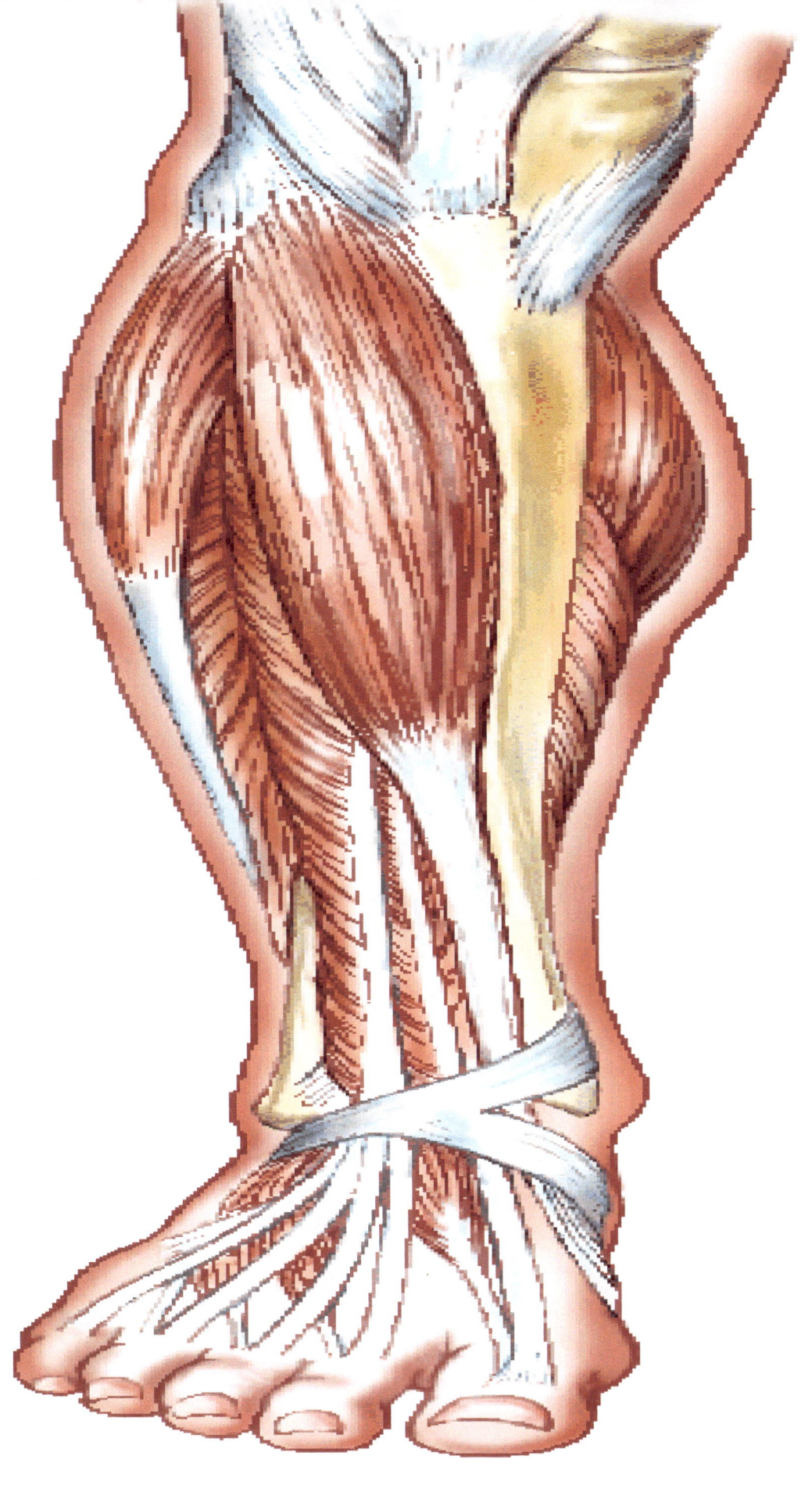

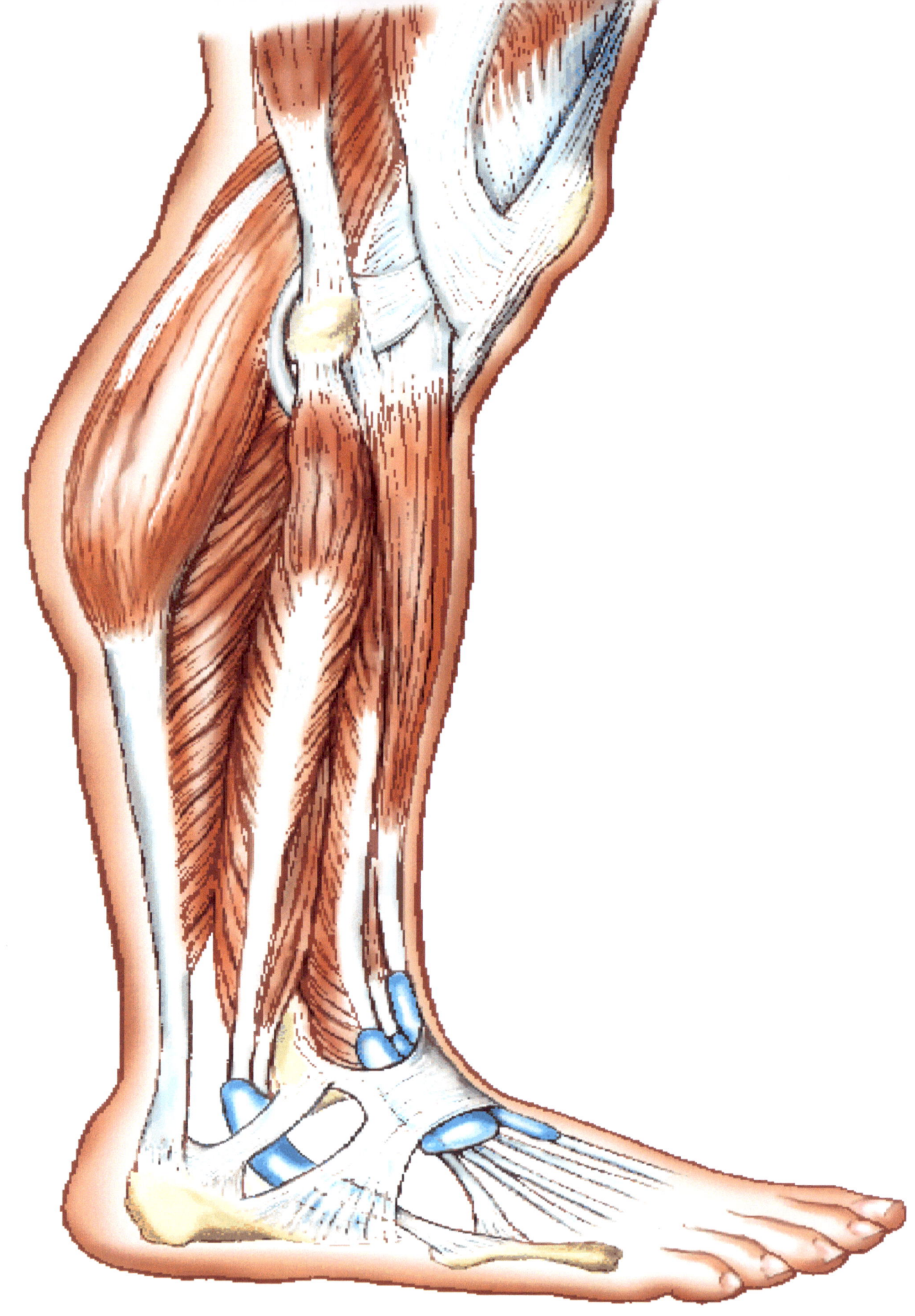

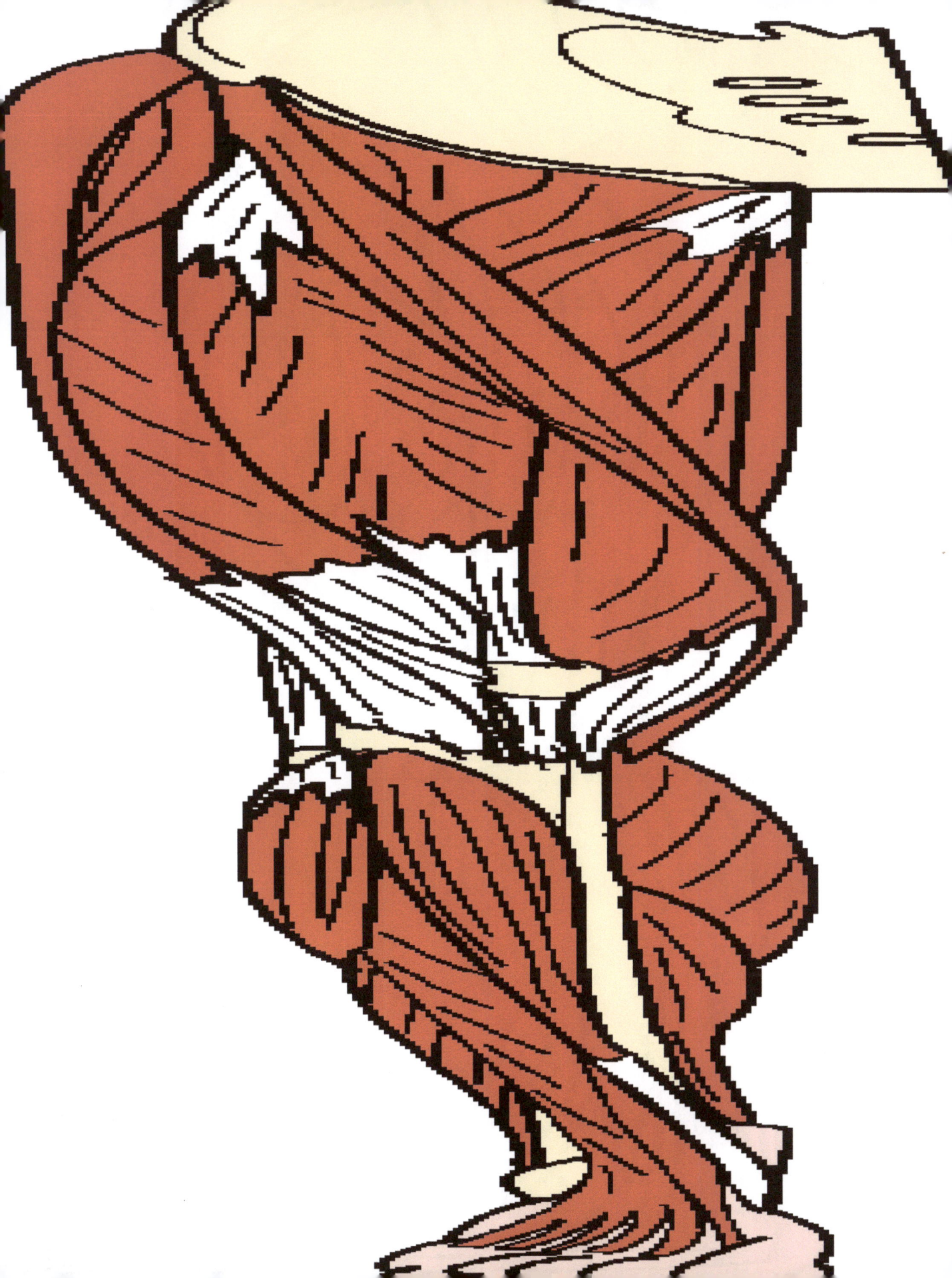

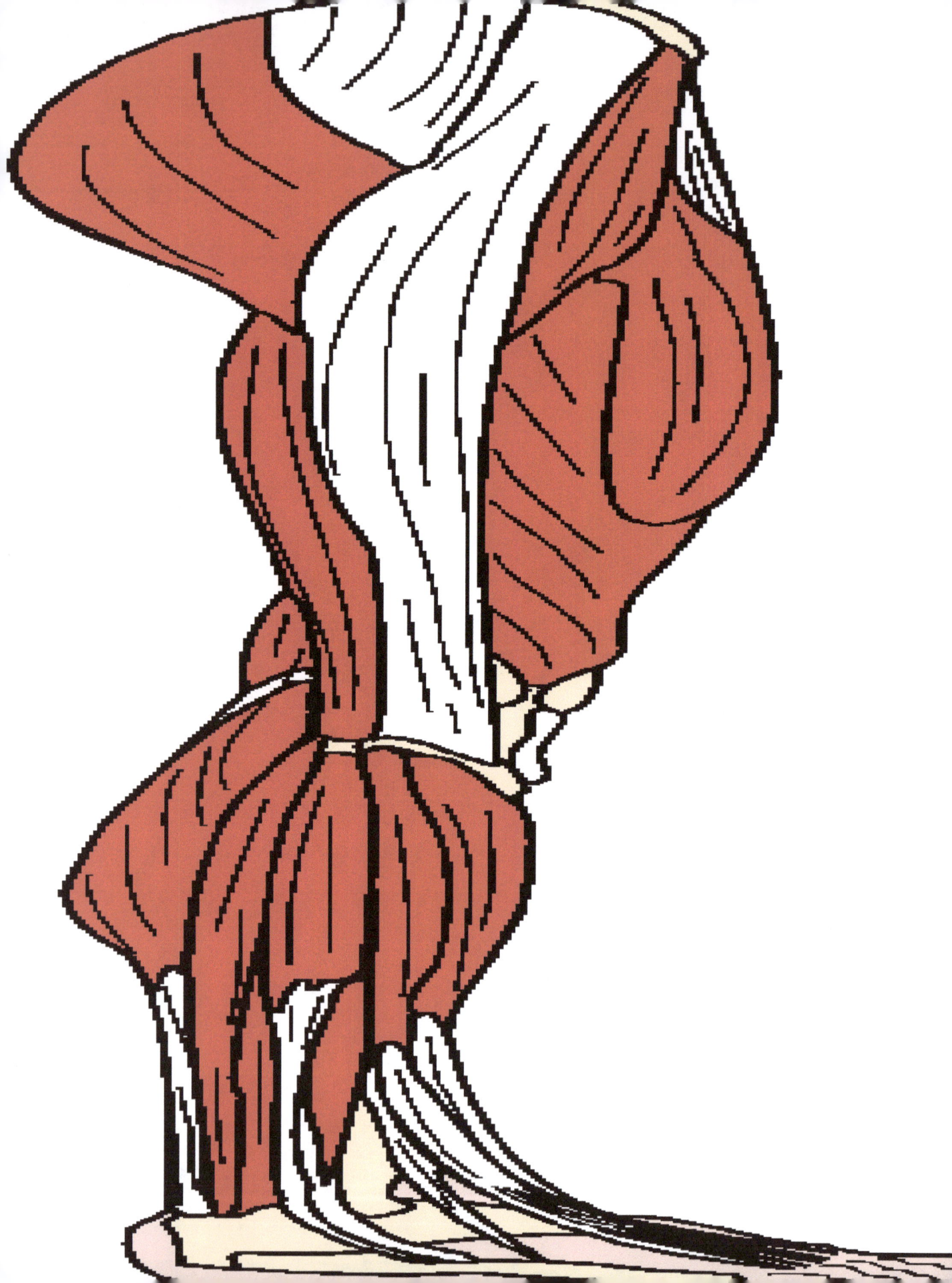

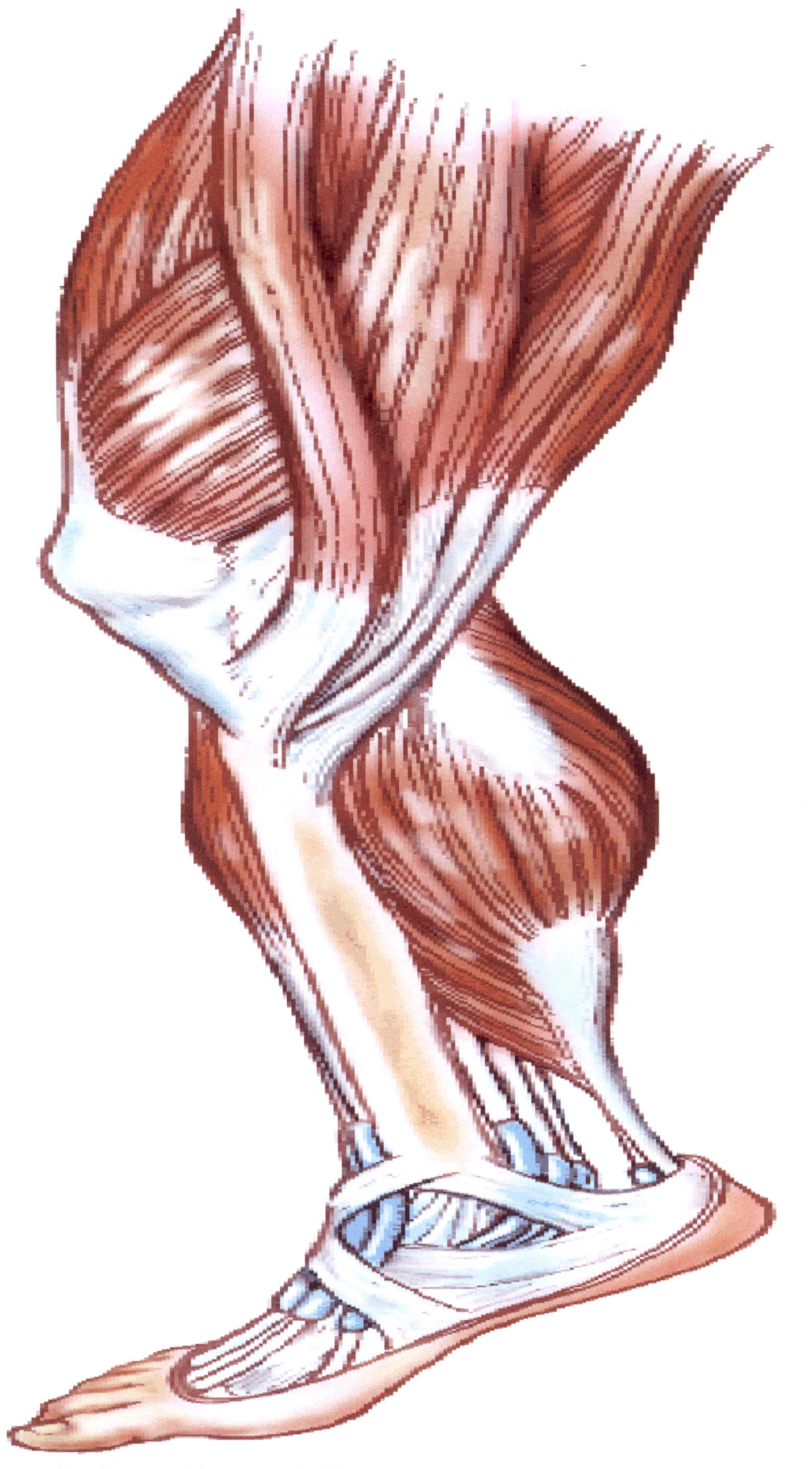

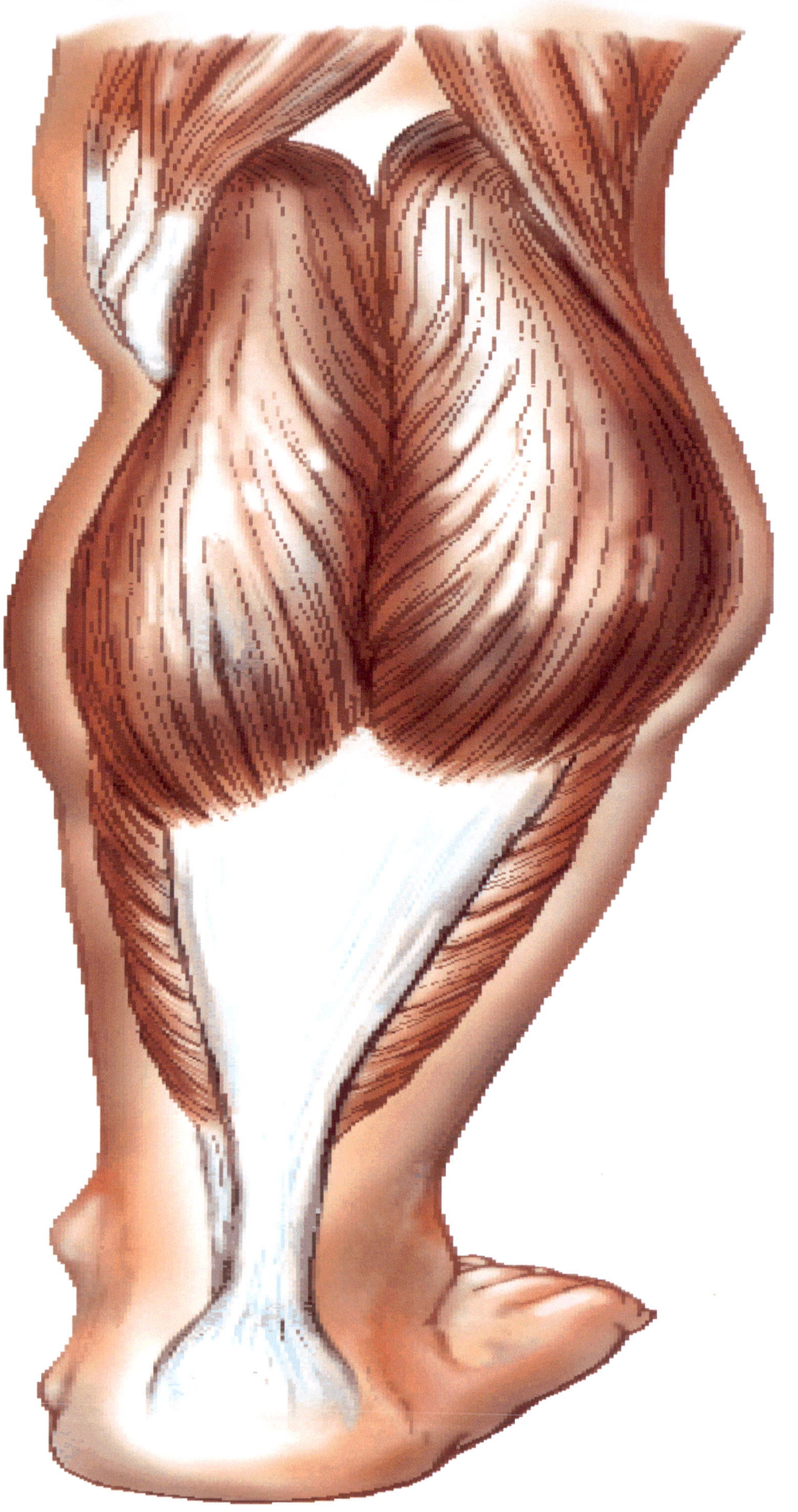

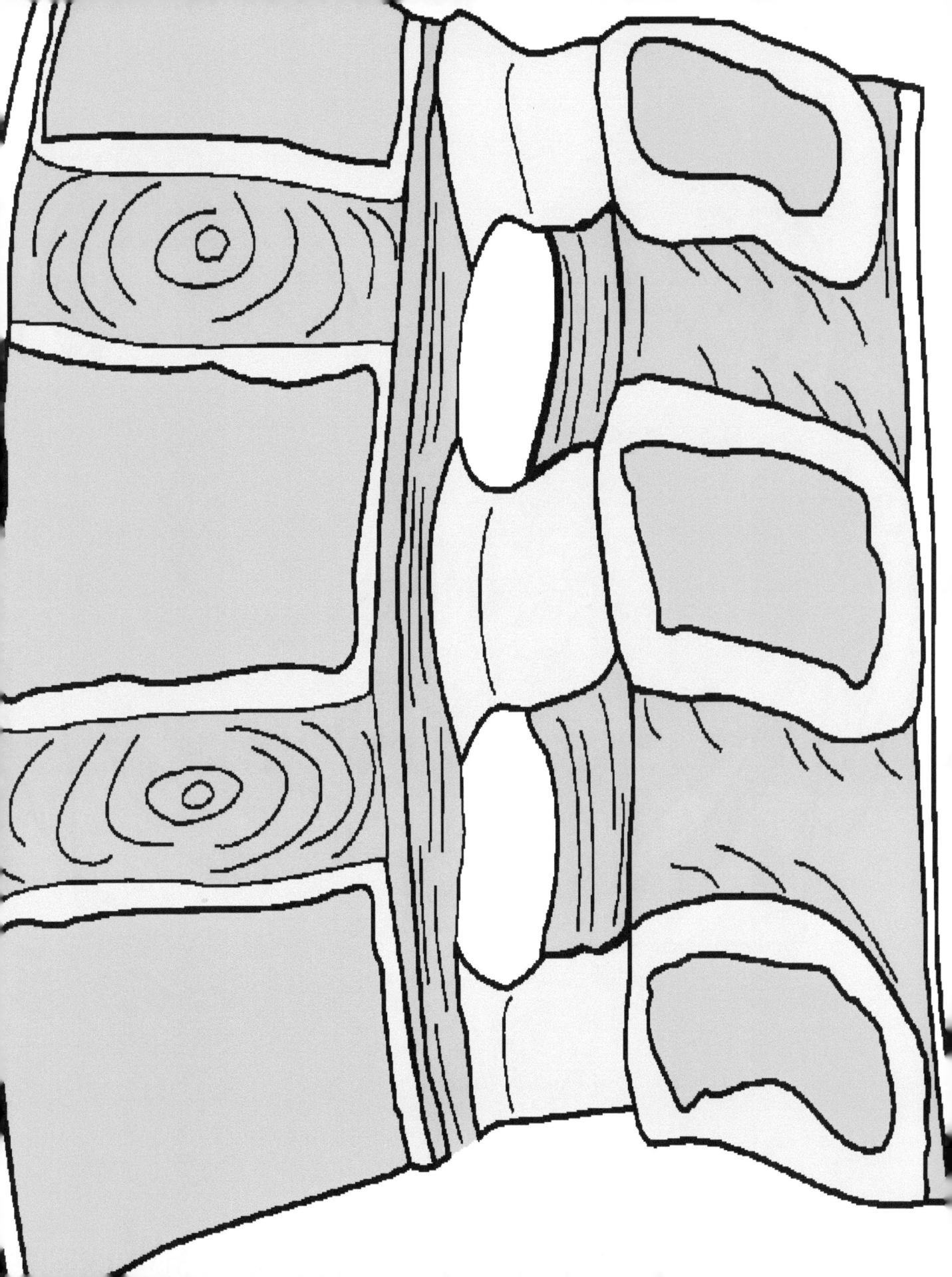

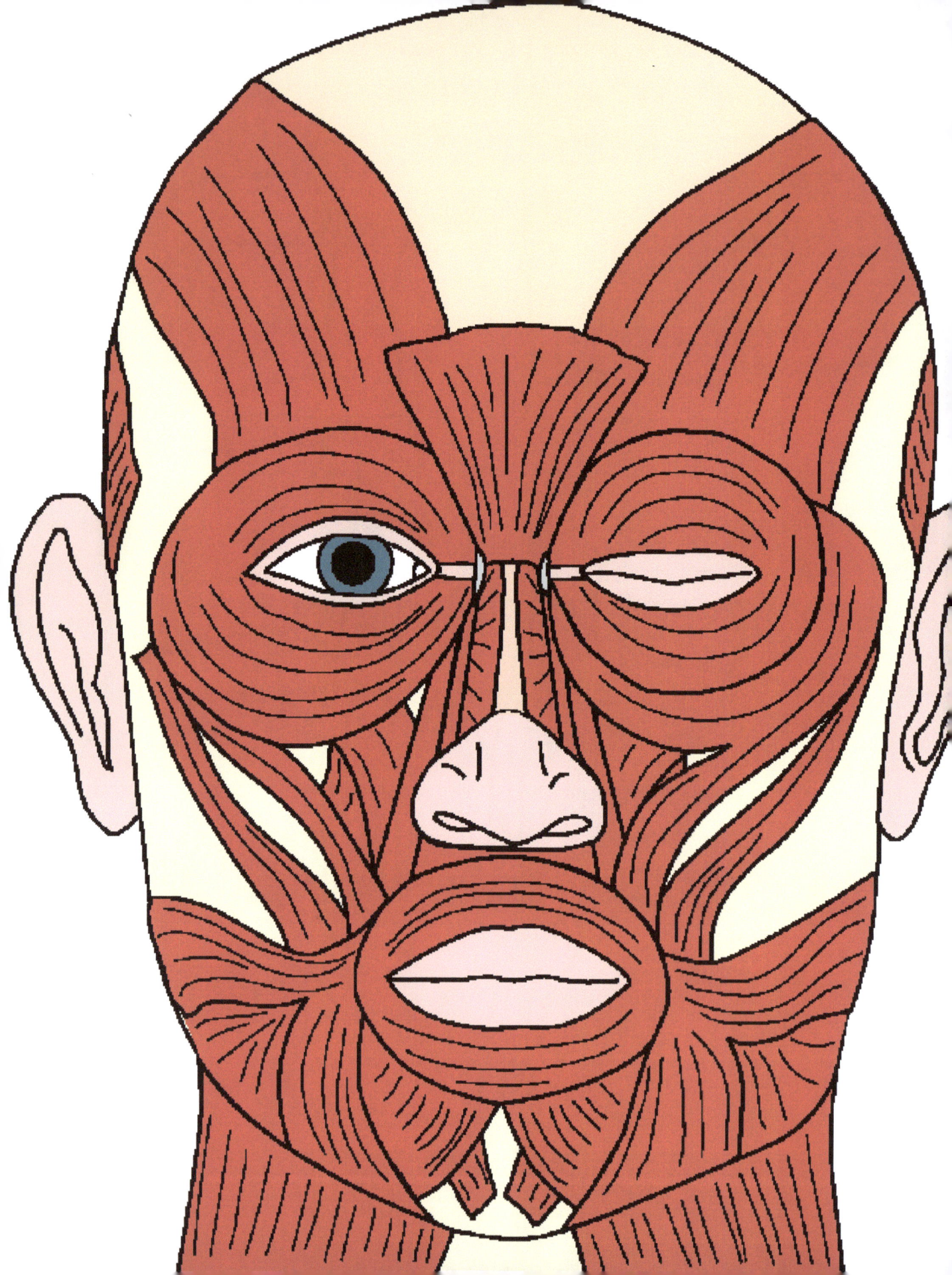

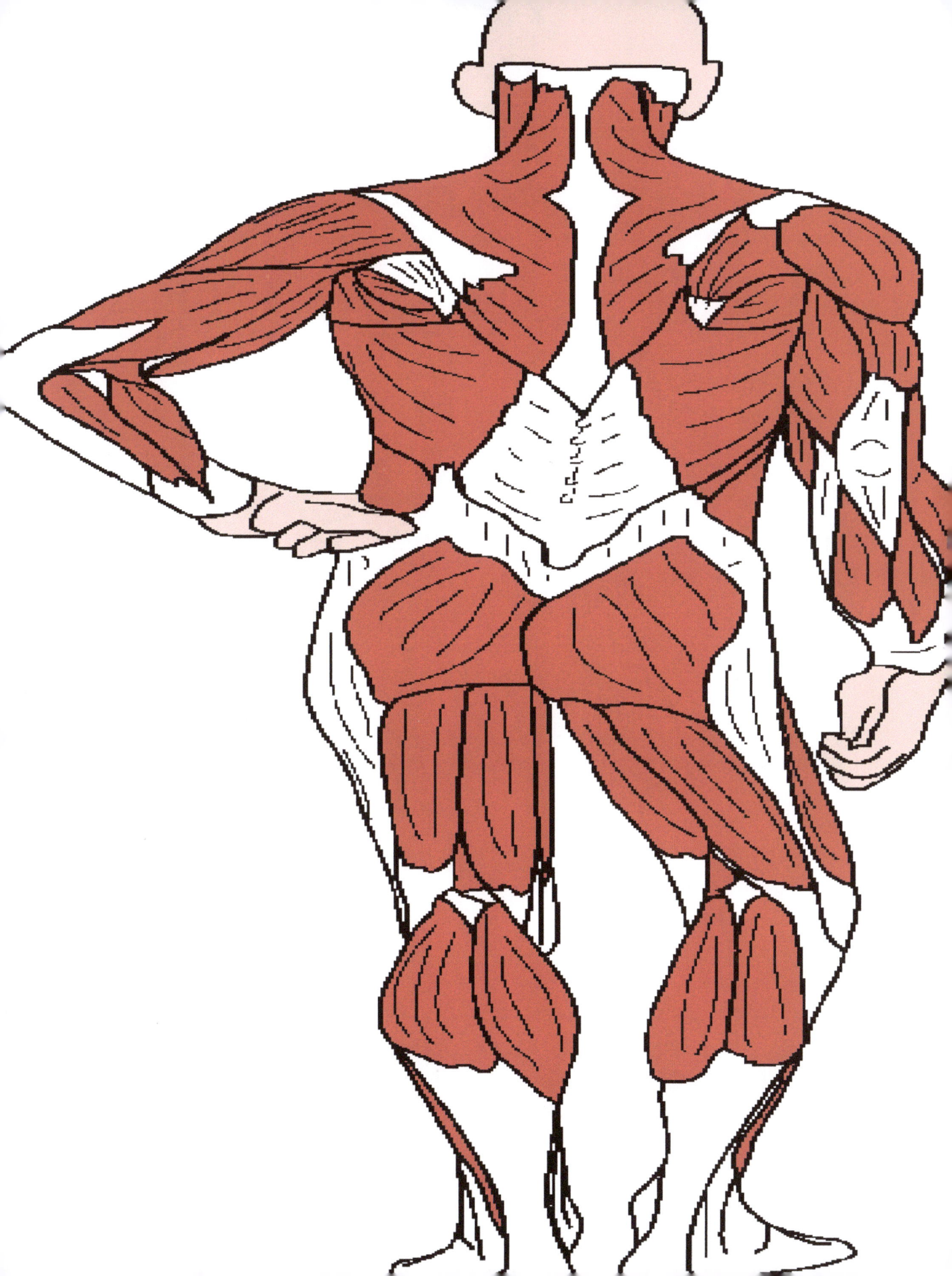

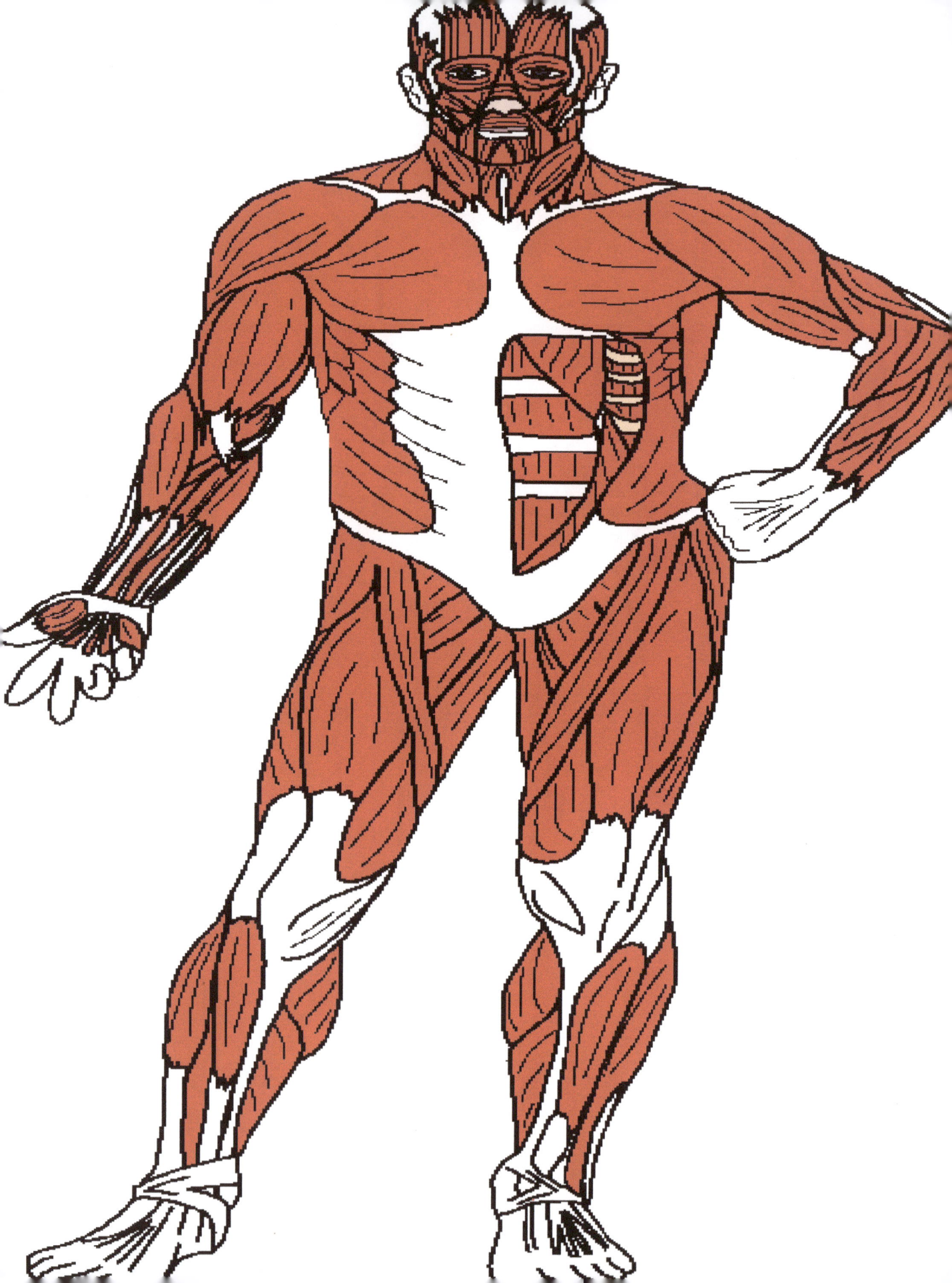

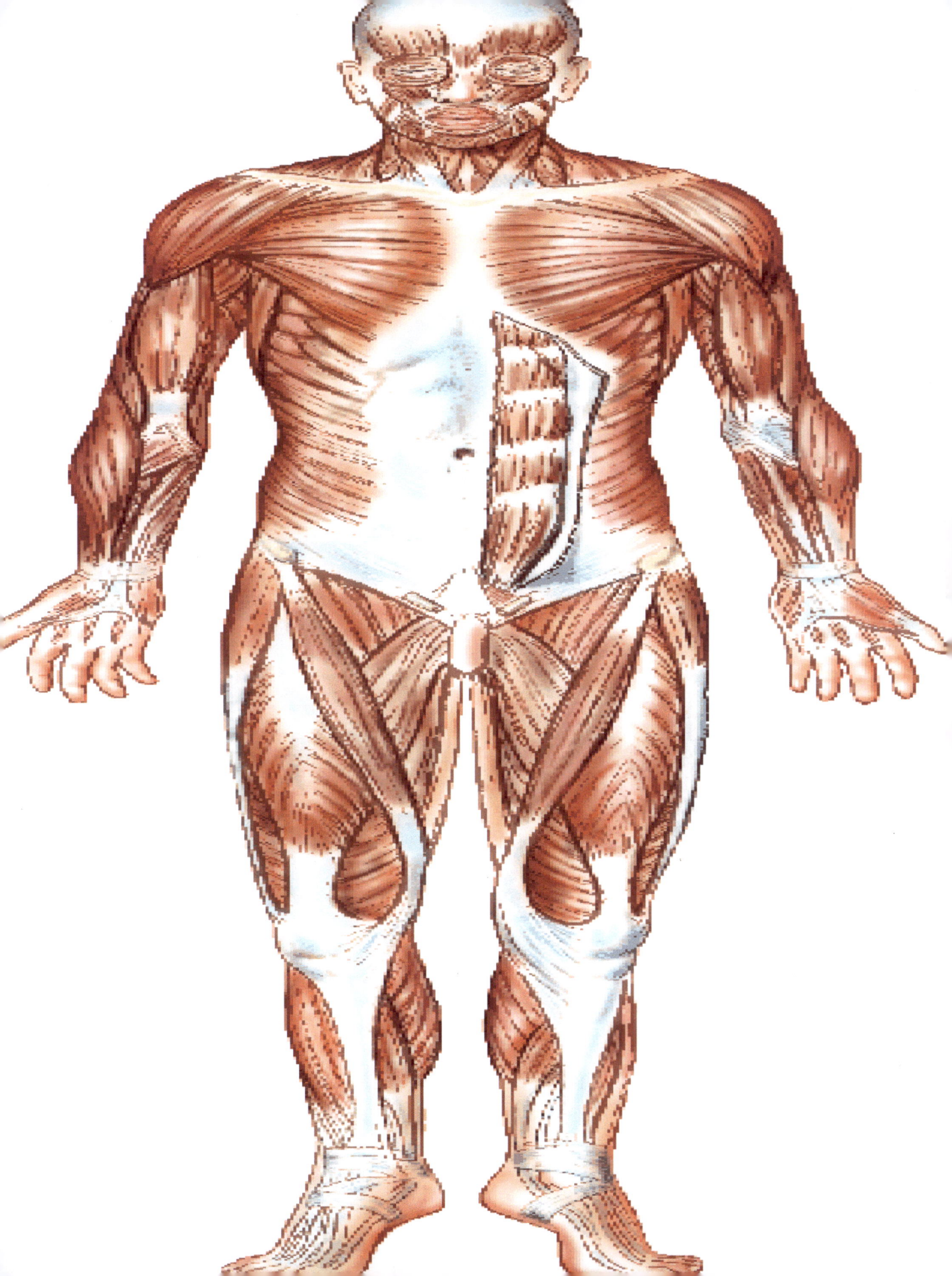

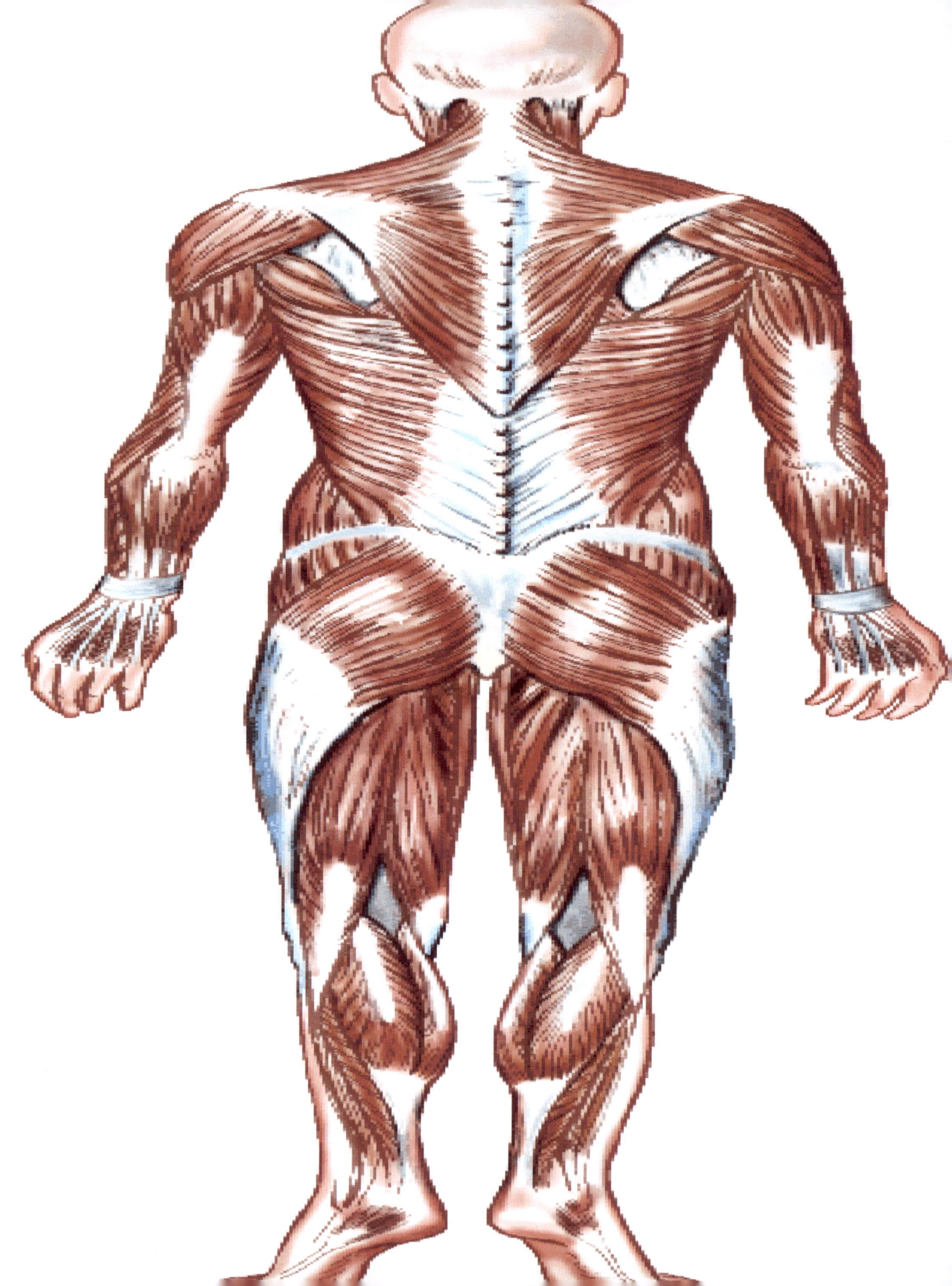

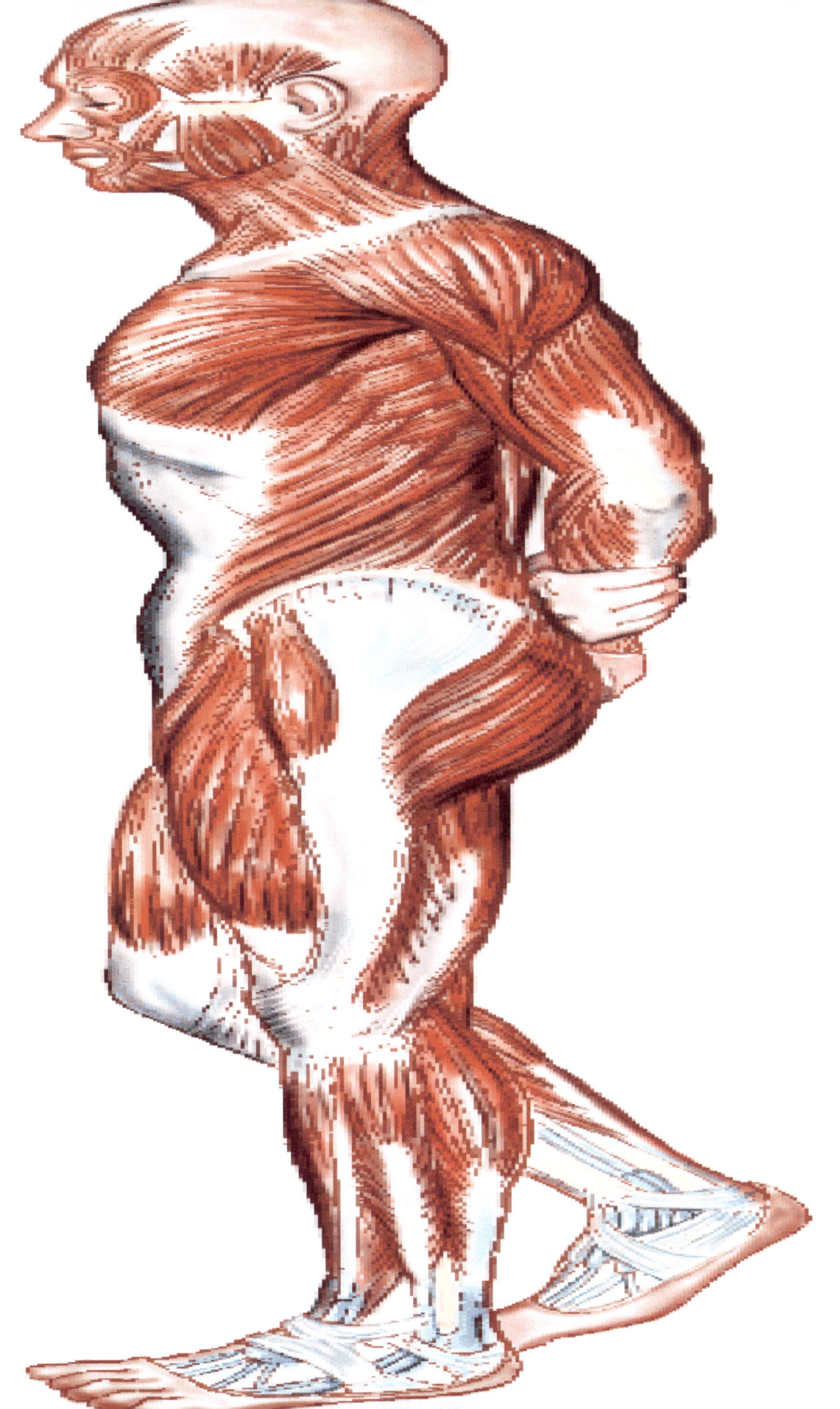

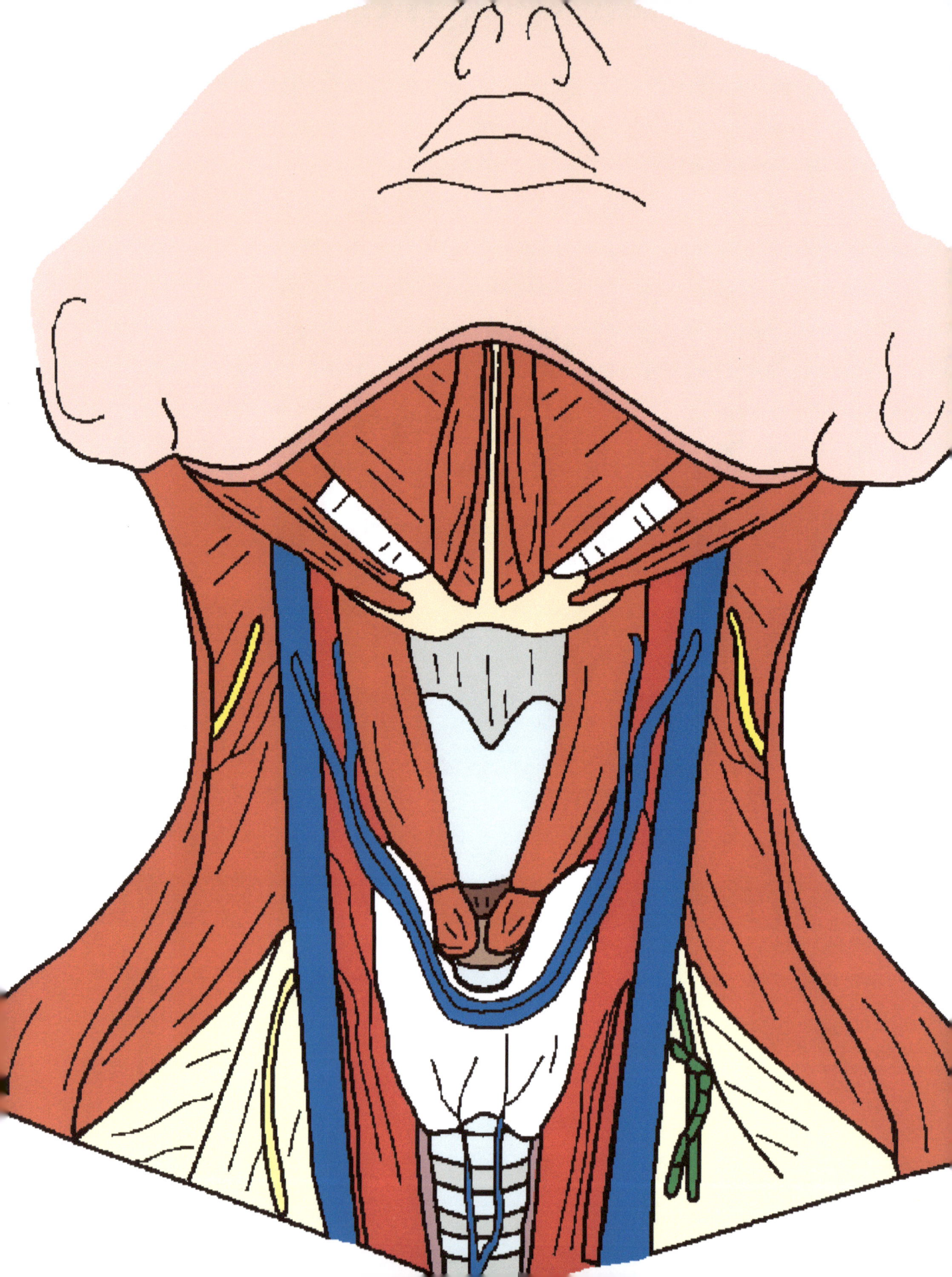

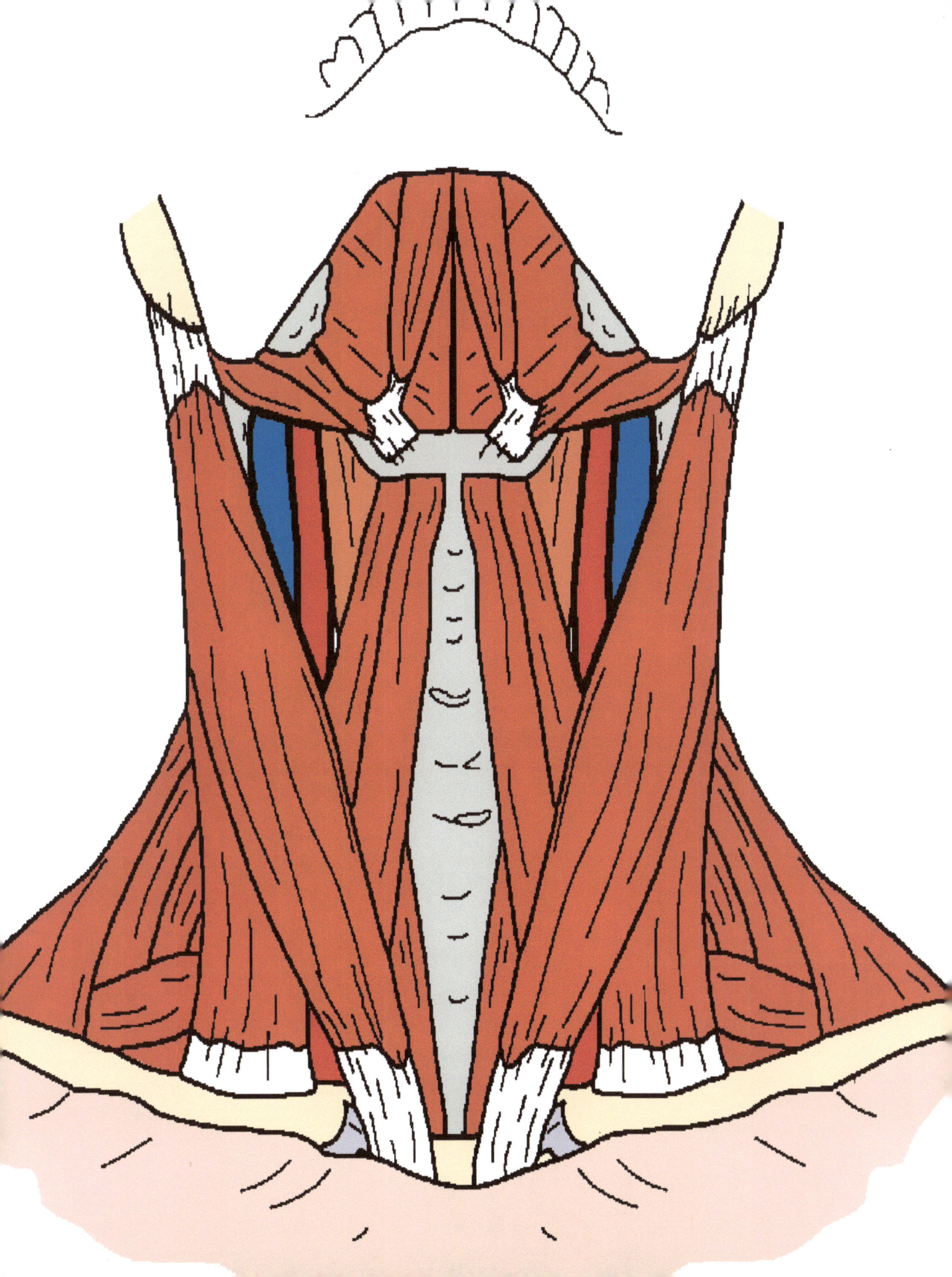

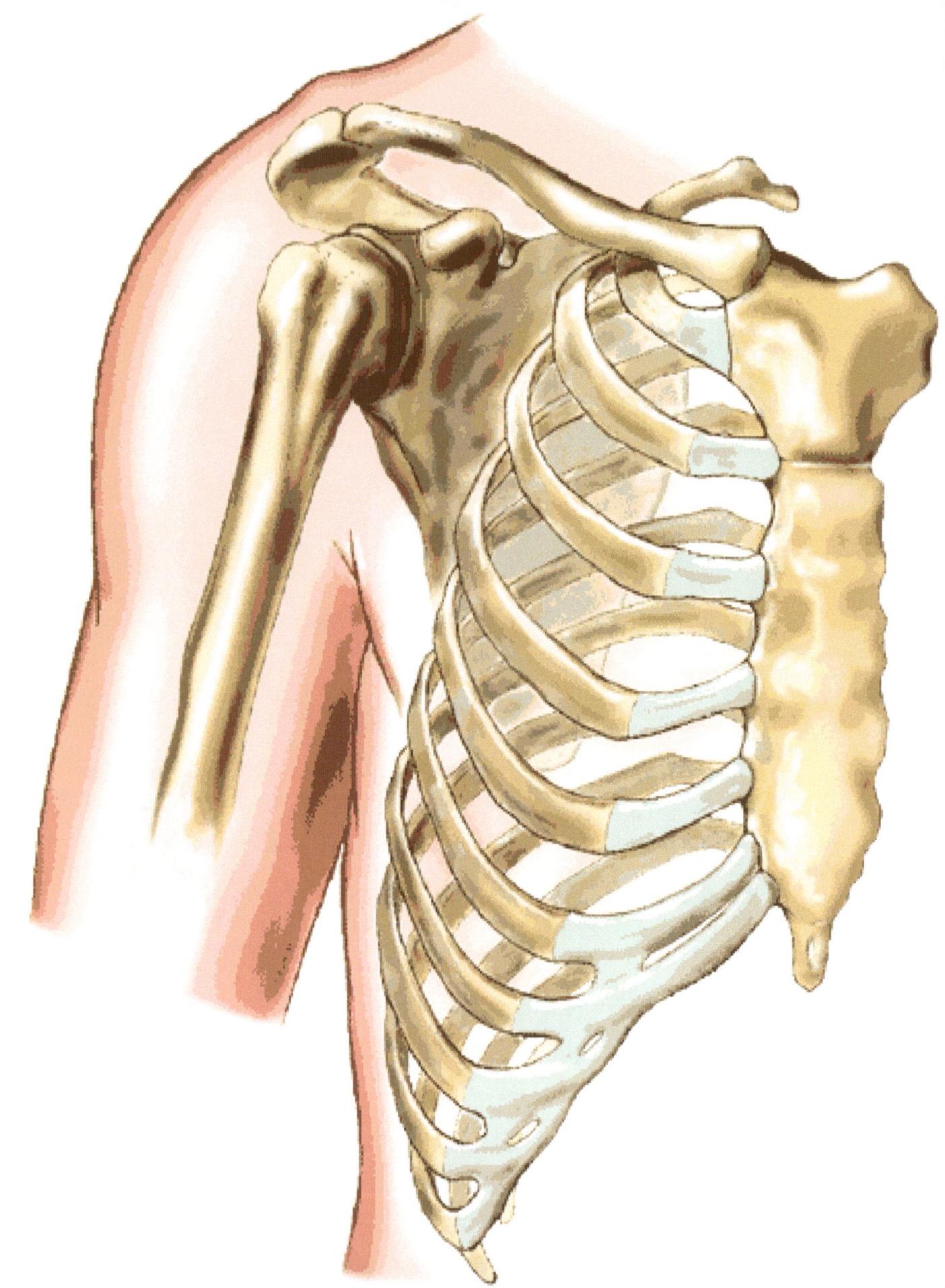

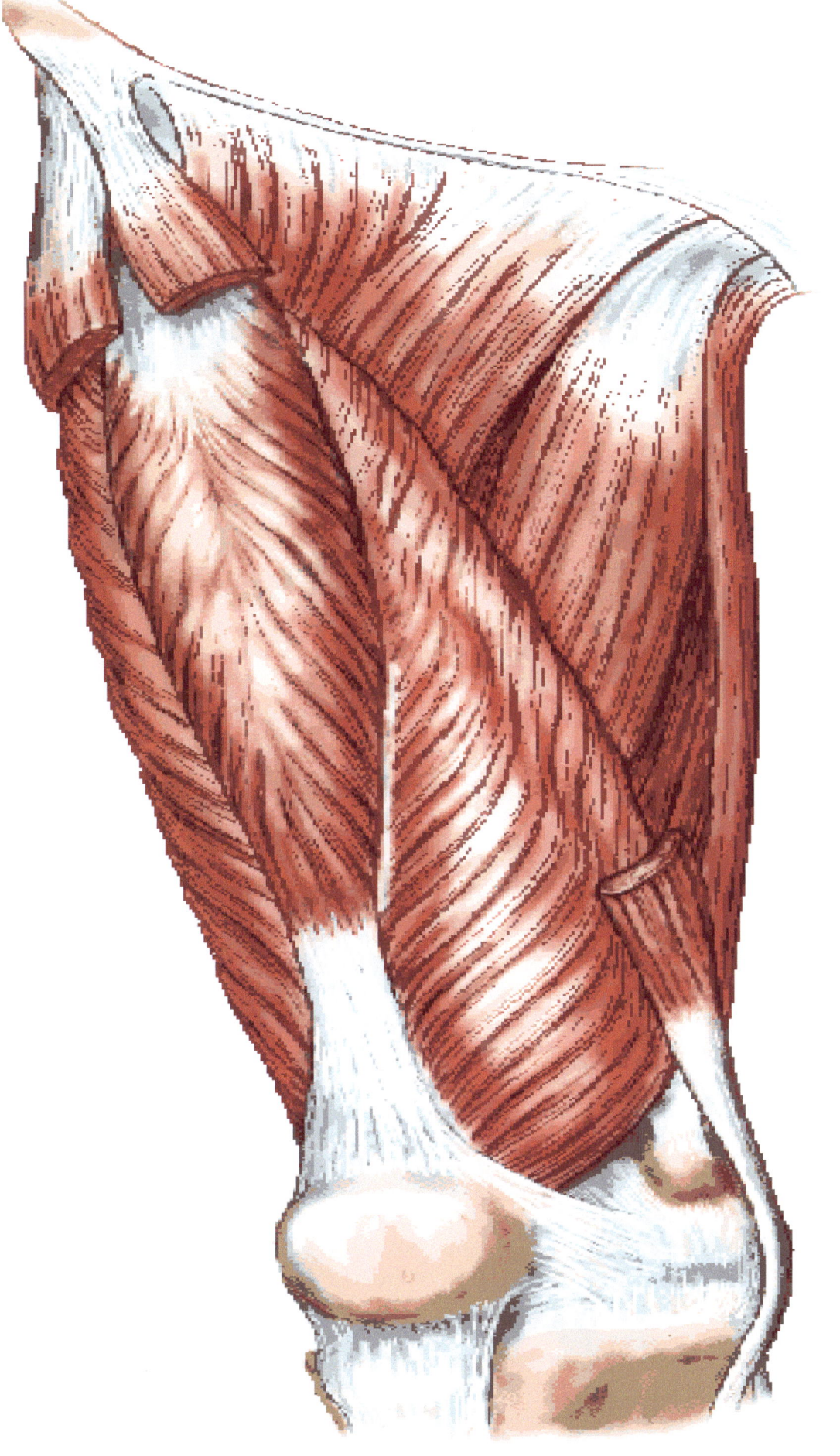

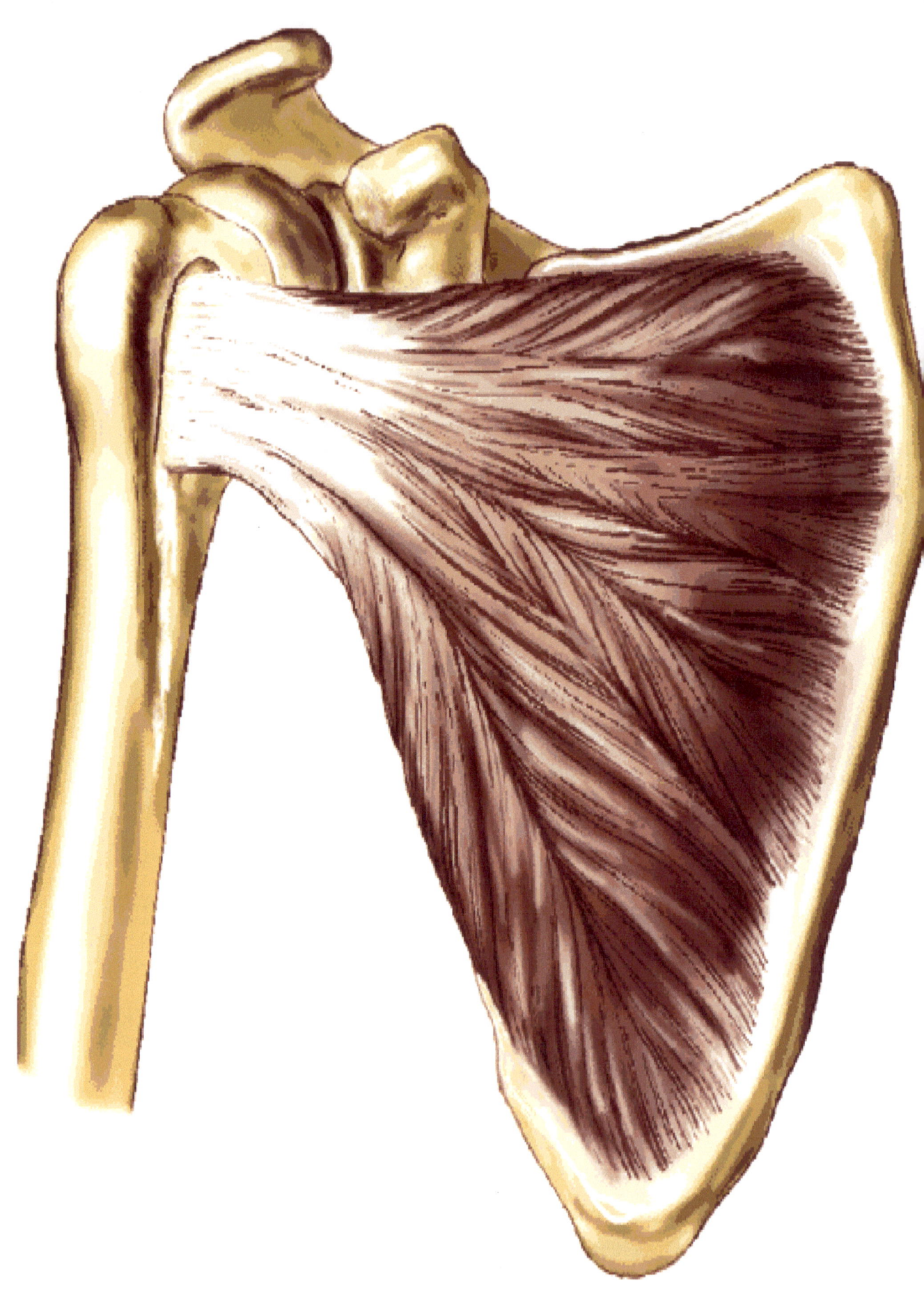

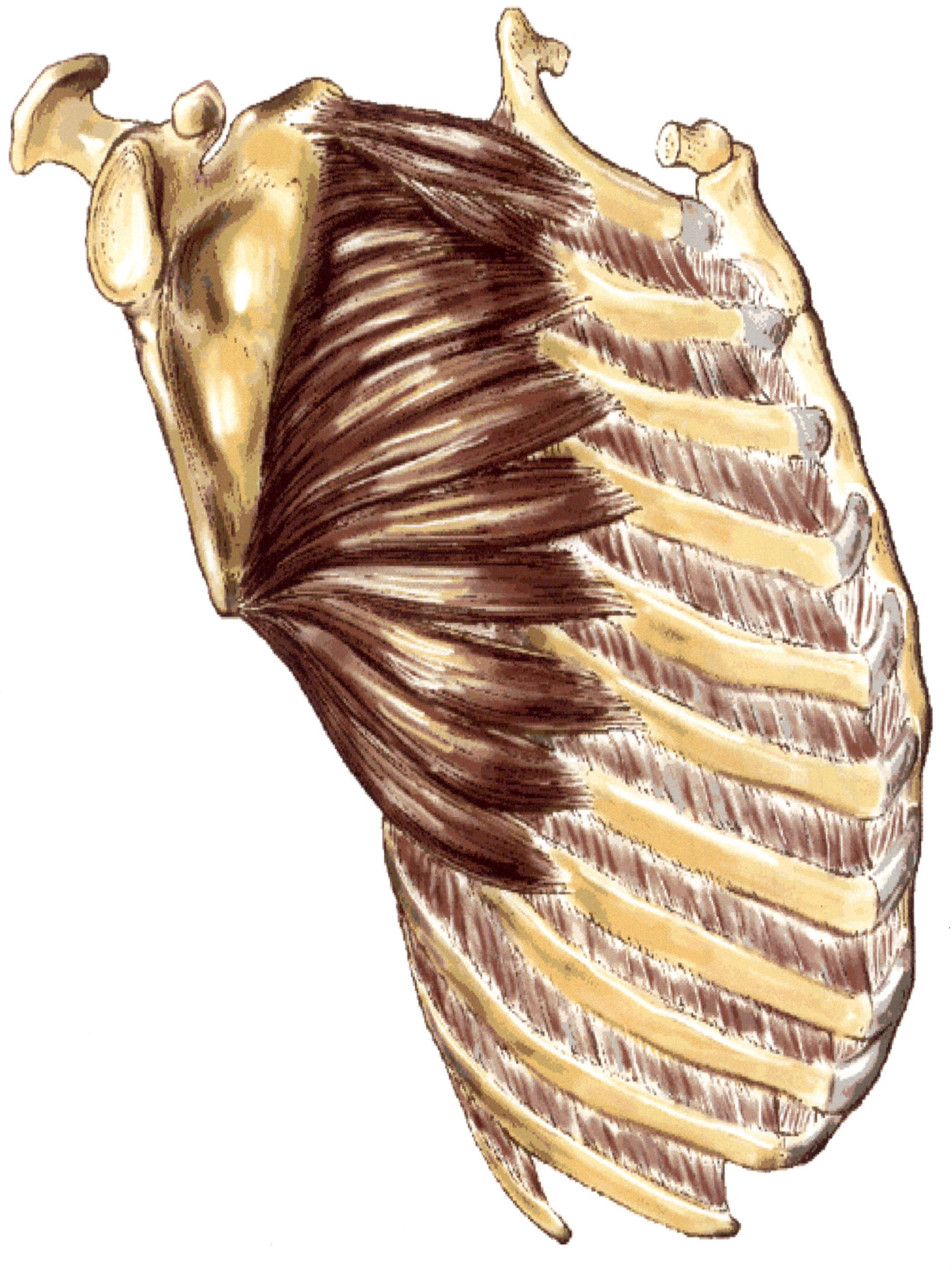

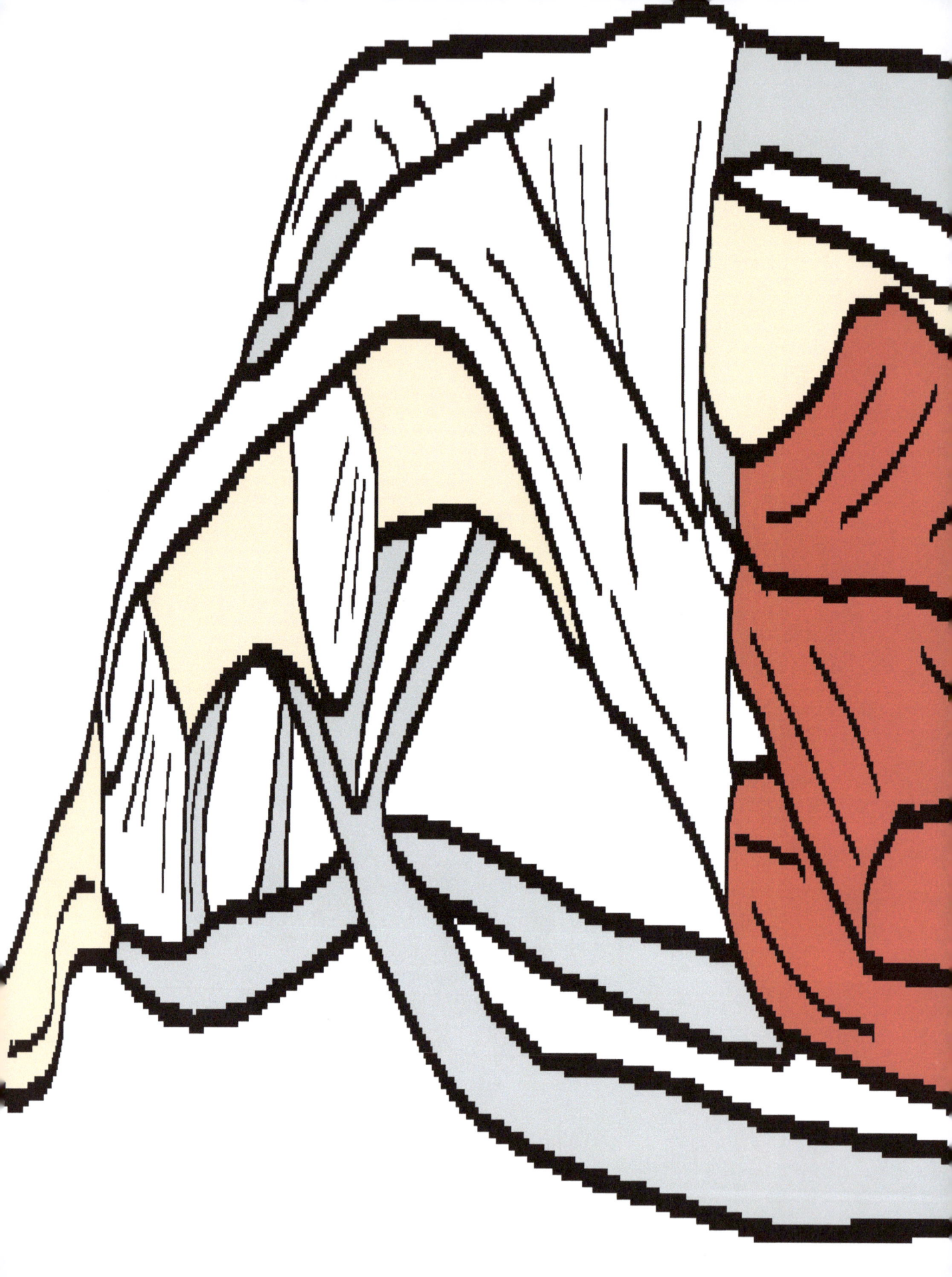

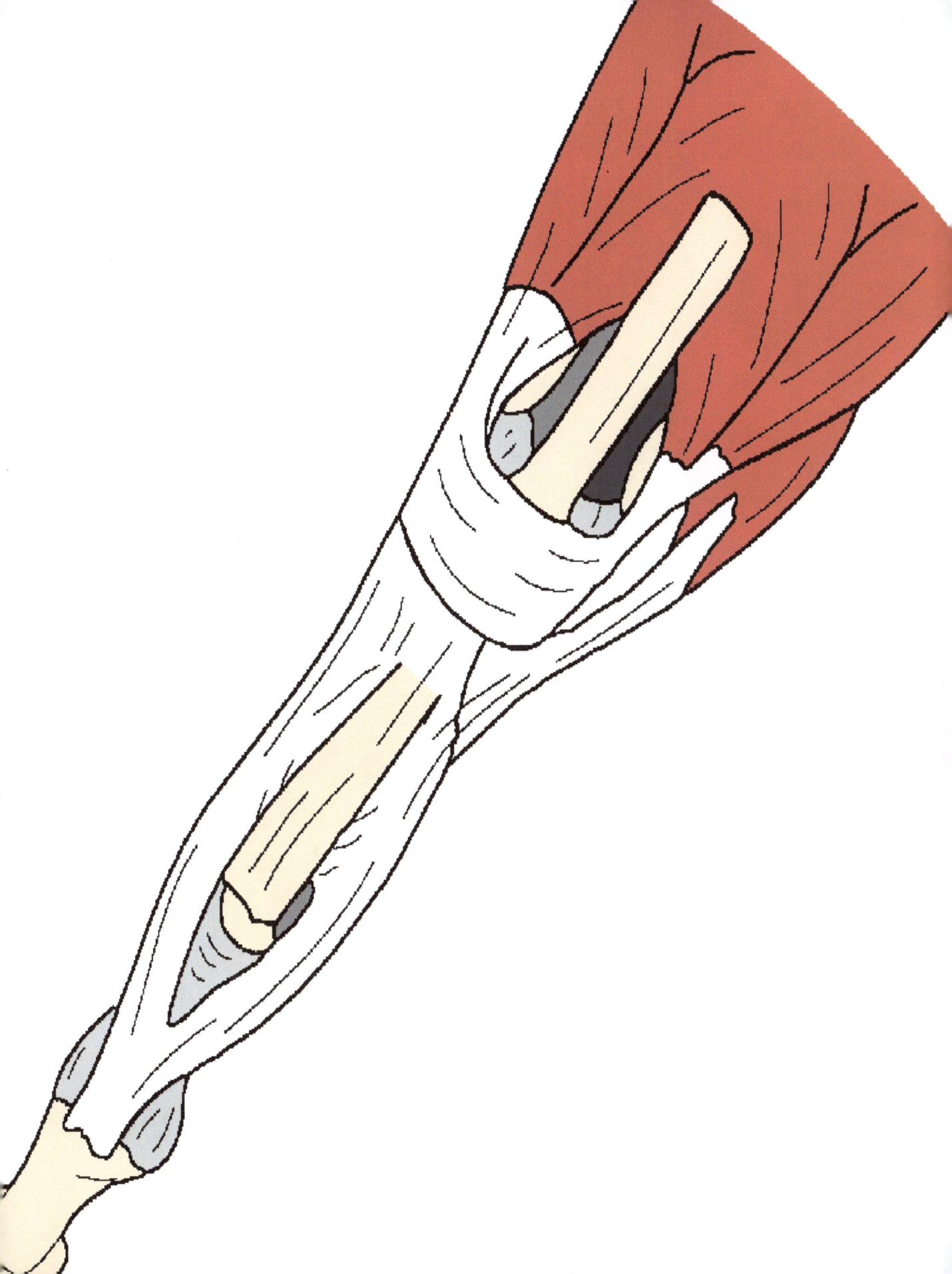

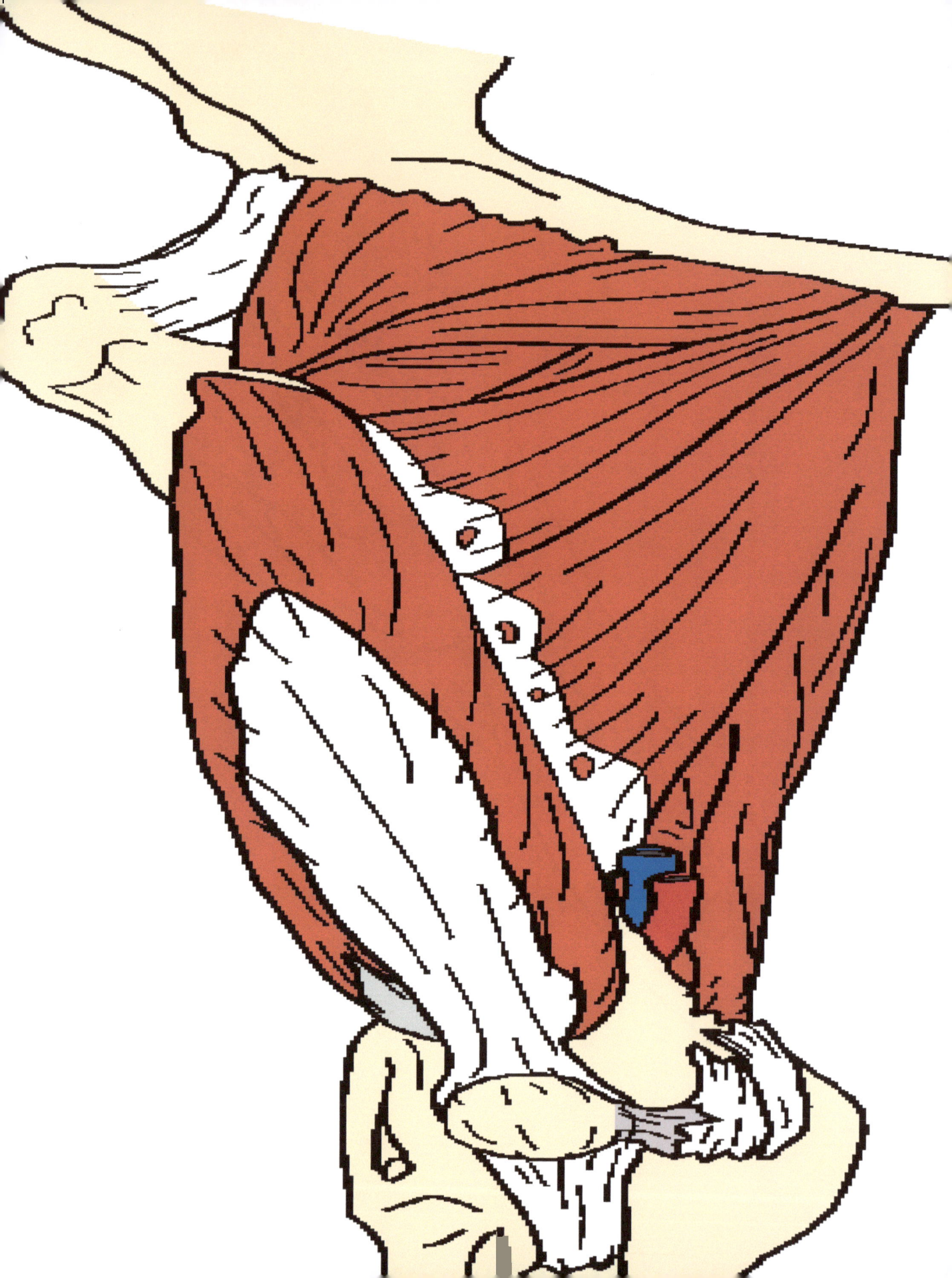

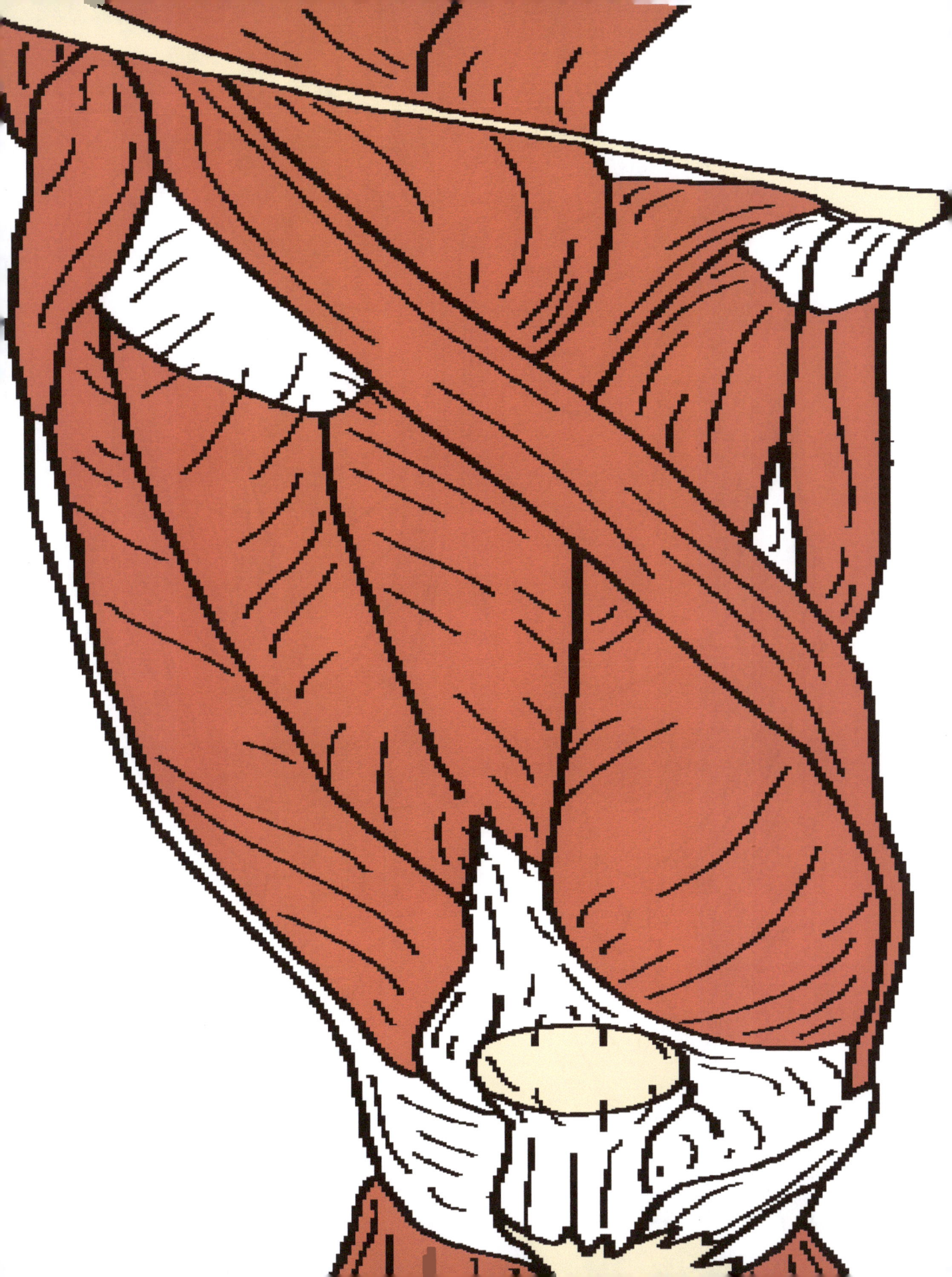

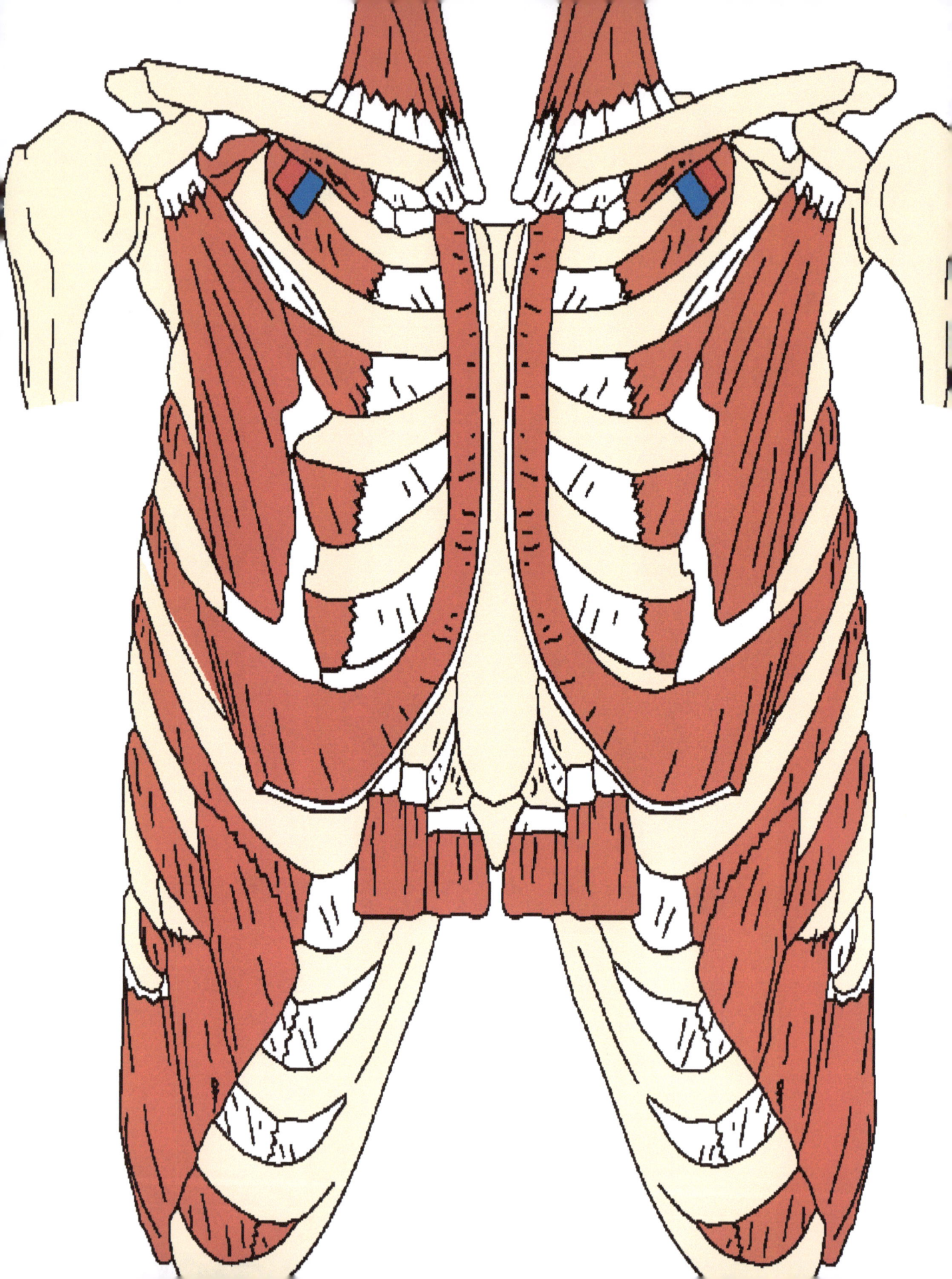

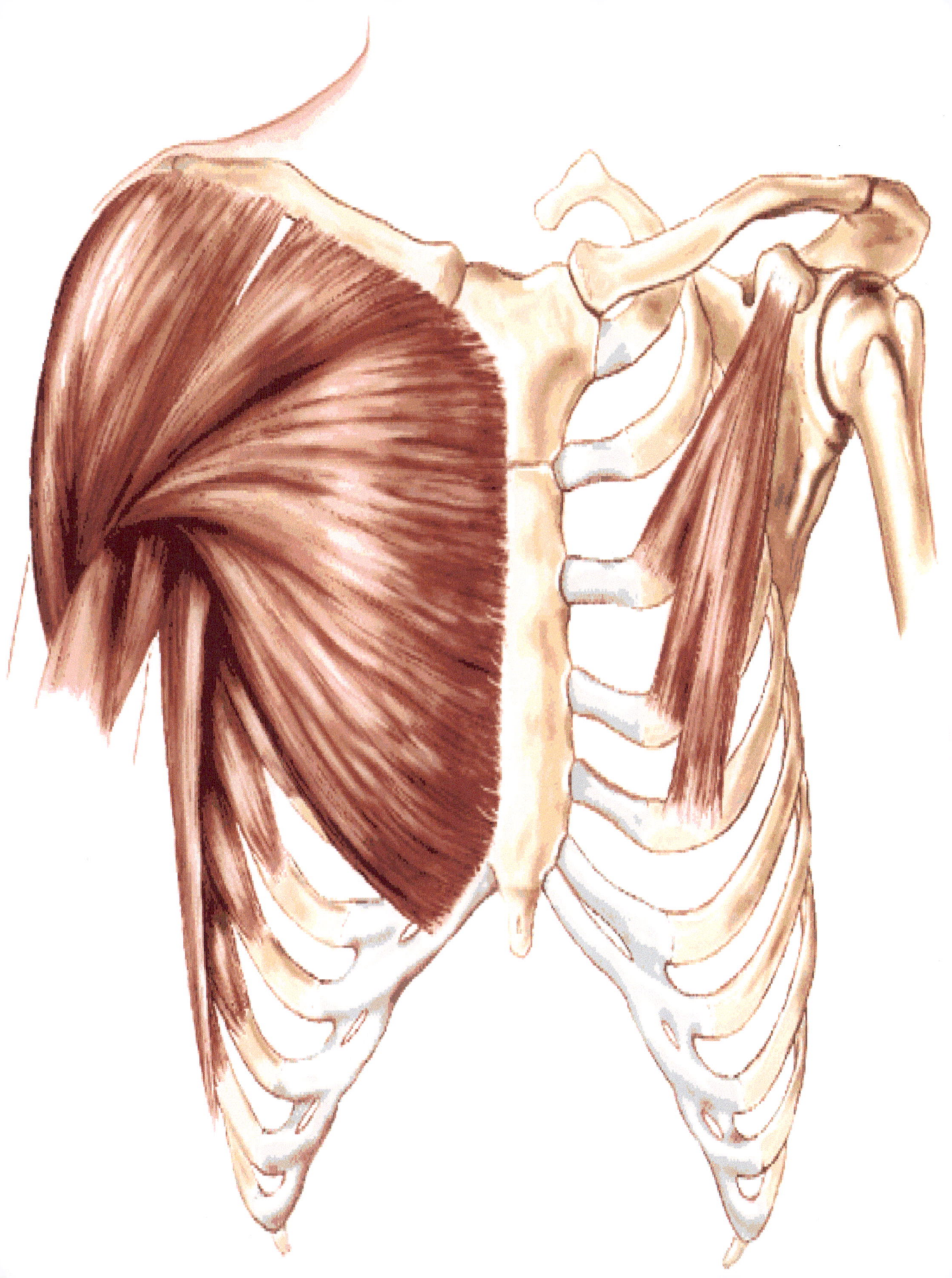

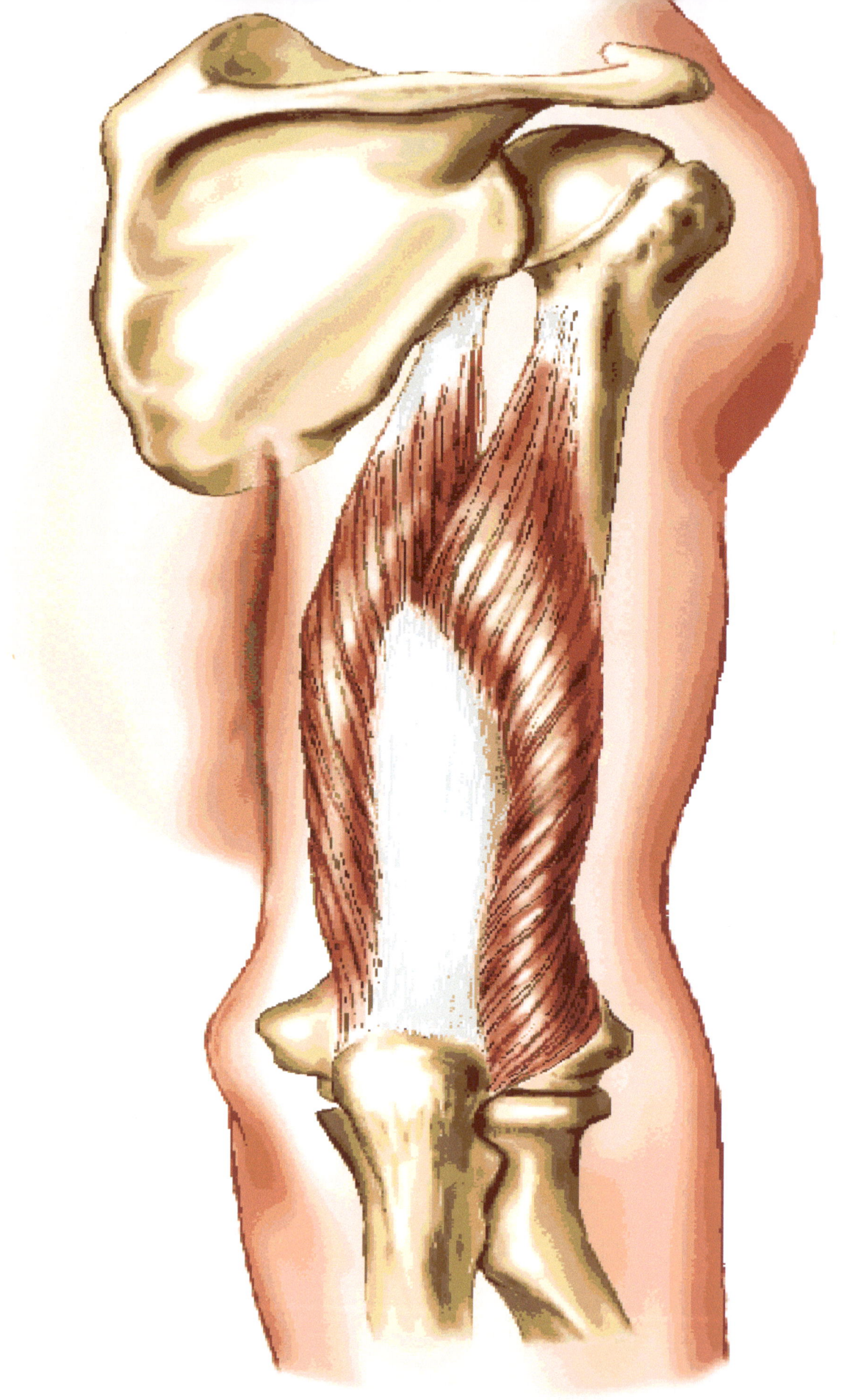

Other Anatomy System Label Practice Books Available on Amazon

1. Cardiovascular System
2. Digestive & Endocrine System
3. Muscular System
4. Nervous System
5. Respiratory System
6. Skeleteal System
7. Surface Anatomy & Senses
8. Urogenital System

www.ingramcontent.com/pod-product-compliance
Lightning Source LLC
Chambersburg PA
CBHW050742180526
45159CB00003B/1324